THE EVIDENCE ROOM

Investigative Case Studies

**A collection of true crime stories of rape and
murder that were eventually solved**

Edited by

RAJU NANDHAKUMAR

Professor of Chemistry

Division of Physical Sciences

*Karunya Institute of Technology and Sciences
(Deemed to be University),*

Karunya Nagar, Coimbatore – 641 114

TamilNadu, India.

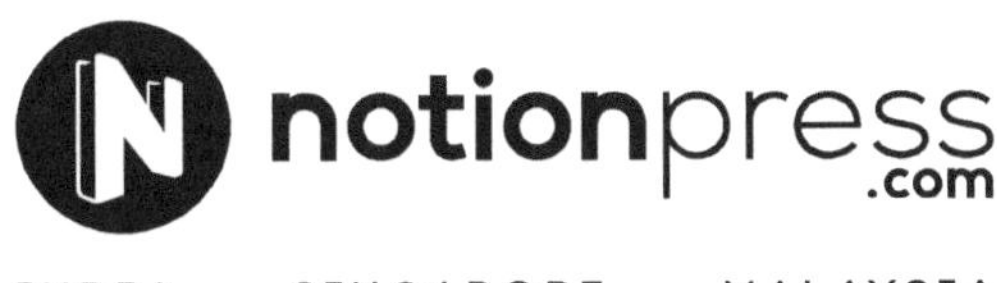

INDIA • SINGAPORE • MALAYSIA

Paperback 979-8-89724-231-3
Hardcase 979-8-89724-232-0

CONTENTS

PREFACE

In the pursuit of justice, Forensic Science plays a vital role in unravelling the mysteries of crime. In the shadows of our society, a sinister reality lurks, shattering the lives of countless individuals and families. This book delves into the darkest corners of human nature, presenting a comprehensive case study of rapes and murders that have left an indelible mark on our collective conscience.

Through meticulous research and a sensitive approach, we aim to shed light on the complexities surrounding these heinous crimes, exploring the motivations, circumstances, and consequences that define them. By examining the intricate web of factors that contribute to such atrocities, we hope to spark a deeper understanding and inspire meaningful dialogue.

This book is not just a chronicle of tragedy, but a call to action – a plea for heightened awareness, empathy, and collective responsibility. May the stories shared within these pages serve as a catalyst for change, ultimately contributing to a safer, more compassionate world for all.

FROM THE EDITOR'S DESK

As the editor of this book on the investigative case studies, I am proud to present a comprehensive resource that summarises some of the complex and sensitive topics of rape and murder inquiries. This book represents the collective expertise of renowned forensic scientists, investigators, and legal professionals who have utilised their knowledge and experience to solve cases.

Our aim is to provide a thorough and objective exploration of the Forensic Science principles and practices applied in these critical cases. We have ensured that the content is accurate, and accessible, making it an invaluable tool for researchers and Students of Forensic Science and related fields.

This book gives an idea about the entire spectrum of Forensic Science disciplines, from crime scene investigation and evidence collection to laboratory analysis and courtroom presentation. We have included real-world case studies, illustrations, and photographs to enhance understanding and illustrate key concepts.

I extend my gratitude to the contributors, reviewers, and production team for their tireless efforts in creating this essential reference. I believe this book will contribute significantly to the pursuit of justice and the advancement of Forensic Science.

Disclaimer: "The views and opinions expressed in these essays are the product of the Forensic Science students' research and discussion involved in its creation. We acknowledge that the content may potentially be sensitive or controversial, and we apologise if any information inadvertently causes offence or discomfort to any individual or group."

Chapter 1

BURGLARY UNCOVERS MURDER SCENE - DNA EVIDENCE REVEALS THE IDENTITY

Rohith Sugu S, Beula M, and Bitto K

ABSTRACT

The crime scene is the most crucial location in any criminal conduct. It is a starting point for criminal investigations, and many clues may have been discovered there. In court, the investigating agency must demonstrate that a crime occurred at a specific location and that physical evidence acquired from that location establishes the identities of the alleged accuser and victim/deceased. It is founded on Locard's concept, which states that the culprit leaves something at the crime scene and takes something from it with him. As a result, professional crime scene visits are particularly important in horrific crimes. It is usually advantageous to arrive at the crime site as soon as feasible. Physical evidence may degrade or deteriorate if the crime is buried for a few days. However, if a small amount of evidence is discovered and meticulously collected by forensic experts, it can be shown to be valuable in court to provide justice. In the case study reported here, just a few dried droplets of blood and two partially burnt bone bits were retrieved 24 days after the occurrence. The only important pieces of evidence for forensic investigation were the two physical pieces of evidence obtained from the crime site. After successfully extracting DNA from microscopic blood and partially burnt bone fragments, DNA profiling was used to determine the identity of the deceased.

KEYWORDS

Crime scene, Locard principle, DNA profiling, evidence collection, extraction, bone pieces, DNA samples.

THE CASE

History: Crime History

Every day, numerous burglary cases are reported in Maharashtra. Young adolescents are involved in most cases.

Once one crime is concealed, they are unafraid to commit the next. This gives them more courage to do horrible atrocities repeatedly. In one instance, three young boys who committed a burglary were apprehended by police from the local crime section. One of them was under the age of eighteen. Police discovered a video of burning footage in the gallery of the juvenile suspected accused's mobile phone while conducting their investigation. Even they captured the blazing spectacle in a selfie. The selfie featured two more blatant intruders. When they inquired, the youngster informed officers of the true incident, which was shocking.

Prior to quitting his employment as a professor due to alcoholism, the guy was a professor. They disregarded him, as did his relatives.

He began attending the neighbourhood court and filing paperwork in criminal defence cases. He interacted with two of the thieves arrested in the incident. At first, he shared their home with them, but due to his alcoholism, he occasionally turned aggressive. He started yelling at them all the time, and once he even insulted their mother in an aggressive manner. Then they made the decision to murder him. They violently murdered him in his room one day at midnight, then attempted to burn his body there using gasoline, but the neighbour of the room was alarmed by the tremendous amount of smoke that was produced.

To escape from the eyes of the neighbours, they put out the fire after that and took his body, still on the scooter, to a remote riverside. They attempted to burn him with the use of a rubber tyre and gasoline, but his body did not totally burn. They used stones to smash the last of the partially burnt body parts, including the skull and major bones, discarded a few bits of bone in the immediate area and the remainder in a neighbouring river's water. Inside the room where the professor was killed, the floor was cleaned, and some of the walls were painted. They also conducted religious ceremonies there. Now the question was: Why did they break his bones and scatter them around? Those perpetrators were aware that if your identification cannot be established and the body of the victim cannot be located after a murder, neither law enforcement nor the legal system will be able to apprehend you or punish you. They therefore took all necessary precautions to remove any potential proof. To prevent suspicion of the location, they attempted to dispose of the body by burning the already burnt portions and discarding the remaining unburnt bones.

VISIT TO CRIME SCENE

Every crime scene requires a thorough analysis. Six steps are involved, including scene assessment, observation, documentation, search, collection, and analysis. There had already been 24 days since the alleged crime when the accused narrated the incident. Police from the criminal branch requested the assistance of the Forensic Science laboratory since the alleged perpetrator took great care not to leave any indication of the horrible crime and because evidence must be gathered through legitimate scientific procedures.

SEARCHING OF CRIME SCENE

To assist the police, a team of forensic specialists went to the crime scene. It was immediately clear that crime scene investigations needed to be conducted in certain steps to prove the linkage idea between the deceased, the accused, the crime scene, and the physical evidence. A bloodstain was frequently discovered as crucial proof of the accused's involvement.

A locked chamber was the first scene. It was split into two pieces after being opened. A large one used as a hall and a smaller one as a kitchen. Between them was a door that opened in the middle. Both side walls near the door looked to be freshly painted. An auspicious term and a religious symbol were engraved in Marathi on the hall's left wall. This made it abundantly evident that there had recently been a religious service there. The ground was cleansed. The floor in the kitchen had some scorched areas. That suggested that there had been a fire there. The kitchen's two walls had little red dots on them. They had a diameter of between 0.2 and 0.3 mm. Instead of swabbing certain places, scraping was used because there was a chance of disturbing the evidence on the cotton swab. As there was a risk of disturbing the evidence on a cotton swab, scraping of such places was used instead of swabbing. A small amount of scraping was analysed for blood using the phenolphthalein reagent. The blood test was positive, and four scraping samples were taken.

The forensic team arrived at crime site number two, which was near the river and slightly distant from scene number one. No one was observed within 500 metres of the home, which was 1.5 kilometres distant. Something looked to have burnt down underneath the Neem tree a few days ago. The suspected accuser stated that this was the location where the dead were burnt. A few completely charred bone bits were discovered after thorough inspection. Then, with the assistance of police officers, a grid search of the surrounding crime scene was conducted. Then they discovered two partially burnt bone fragments.

ANALYSIS OF EVIDENCE

The investigation agency sent over the material to the Regional Forensic Science Laboratory in Nashik. DNA profiling was performed on the extracted samples.

EXTRACTION OF DNA

The process of extracting DNA from a material by physical and/or chemical means is known as DNA extraction. It involves separating DNA from biological components such as proteins and cell membranes. Friedrich Miescher achieved the first successful isolation of DNA in 1869.

High-quality, pure DNA devoid of contaminants like RNA and proteins should be effectively extracted using DNA isolation methods. Both manual methods and commercially available kits are used for DNA extraction. Many tissues may be used to extract DNA, such as blood, body fluids, frozen tissue sections, formalin-fixed paraffin-embedded tissues, direct fine needle aspiration cytology (FNAC) aspirate, and more. Once the cells have been lysed and the DNA has been dissolved, macromolecules, lipids, RNA, and proteins are extracted using chemical or enzymatic techniques. DNA may be extracted using three different methods: organic extraction (phenol-chloroform technique), non-organic extraction (salting out and proteinase K treatment), and adsorption method (silica-gel membrane).

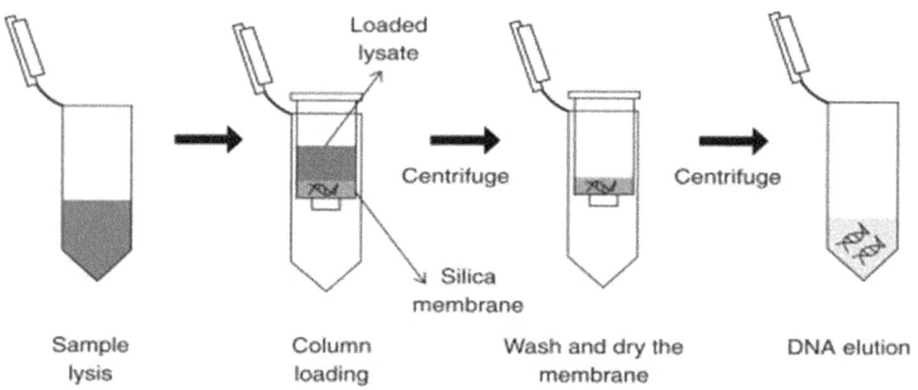

The Column DNA extraction

DNA EXTRACTION FROM BONE

The whole bone powder was subjected to the standard phenol-chloroform procedure (PCE) in accordance with the modified methodology of Hochmeister and Budowle. After digesting bone powder for a full night, phenol-chloroform-isoamyl alcohol was used to extract DNA, which was then purified and concentrated to a volume of 15 µl using microcolumns (Ultracel YM 100, Microcon). In line with *Salamon et al.'s* description, DNA was extracted from bone crystal aggregates (EA). In conclusion, 2.5% NaOCl was added to 500 mg of bone powder and incubated for 4 hours. The particle was centrifuged, rinsed with water and 95% ethanol, resuspended in 100% ethanol, and allowed to dry overnight. After being vortexed and sonicated, the dry material was left to settle in 95% ethanol. Following a few EDTA solution exchanges and centrifugation, the precipitant was subjected to decalcification in 0.5 M EDTA pH 8.0 after being cleaned with 2.5% NaOCl and water. Proteinase K, DTT, EDTA, NaCl, and SDS were added to decalcified bone powder and incubated for 30 minutes at 60°C and overnight at 37°C. By phenol-chloroform-isoamyl alcohol, DNA was extracted, purified, and concentrated by ultrafiltration (Ultracel YM 100, Microcon) to a volume of 15 µl. Total demineralisation (TD) was used to extract DNA in compliance with the *Loreille et al.* methodology. The extraction buffer (0.5 M EDTA, 1% lauryl sarcosyl) and 200 ml of 20 mg/ml proteinase K were added to 500 mg of bone powder, which was then incubated overnight at 56°C. The bone powder was then concentrated using Centricon Plus-20 and filtered using a Centricron thirty centrifugal filter unit (Millipore). Appropriate controls and disinfection procedures were followed at every stage of the extraction process.

ANALYSIS

To extract DNA, scrapings and powder from partly burnt bone pieces were gathered. Five little pieces of scraping were gathered to isolate the DNA. If bone pieces were only partially burnt, the less charred section was selected, and powder was taken out of it. Using the Automate Express machine and the PrepFiler™ Express DNA extraction kit for blood and the PrepFiler™ BTA DNA extraction kit for bone, respectively, DNA was extracted from both blood and bone. One helpful tool for separating DNA from a variety of biological materials is the PrepFilerTM Forensic DNA extraction kit (Applied Biosystems,

Foster City, CA). It was established to know how much DNA had been taken.

PCR TECHNIQUE

The polymerase chain reaction (PCR) is a commonly used method for rapidly producing millions to billions of copies of a given DNA sample, allowing scientists to amplify a very tiny amount of DNA (or a portion of it) sufficiently for extensive investigation. Kary Mullis, an American scientist at Cetus Corporation, devised PCR in 1983. Mullis and biologist Michael Smith, who had invented other crucial methods of altering DNA, shared the Nobel Prize in Chemistry in 1993.

Many processes used in genetic testing and research, such as the study of ancient DNA samples and the identification of infectious organisms, rely on PCR. In a series of temperature adjustments, copies of extremely tiny quantities of DNA sequences are exponentially amplified using PCR. PCR is currently a widespread and frequently required technology in medical laboratory research for a wide range of applications, including biological research and criminal investigations. Denaturation was performed on the DNA samples HiDiFormamide and Liz 600 size standards. Accurately measured DNA was used for PCR amplification using the AmpFlSTR Identifiler PCR amplification kit on an Applied Biosystems Veriti Thermal Cycler. Following PCR amplification, STR DNA profiling was performed effectively on a Gene analyser 3500 equipment. DNA profiles were acquired from scraping and bone parts. Meanwhile, the laboratory obtained blood from the deceased's parents. Blood samples were also DNA profiled using the Gene analyser 3500 equipment.

RESULT OF THE ANALYSIS

DNA profiles acquired from scraped blood and DNA profiles recovered from partially burnt bones were similar and came from the same male source. The profiles were matched to the blood of the claimant. The putative parents matched paternal and maternal alleles found in scraped and partially burnt bone fragments. DNA profiles from two distinct crime locations verified the sequence of events described by the suspect. It also established the deceased's identity.

PICTORIAL REPRESENTATION

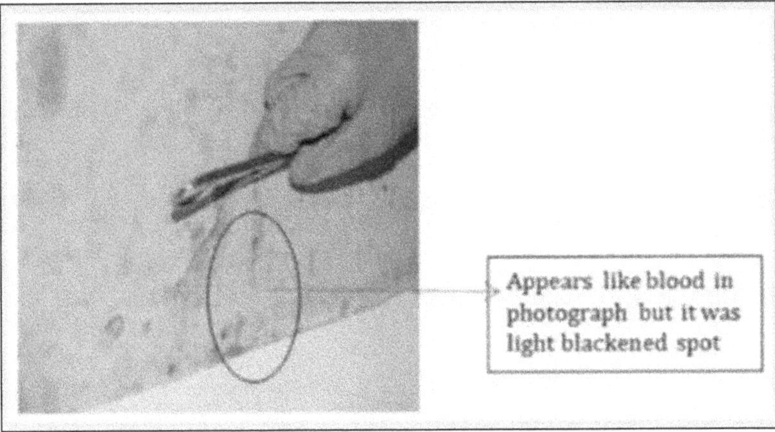

Figure 1 Collection of Scrapping from Wall

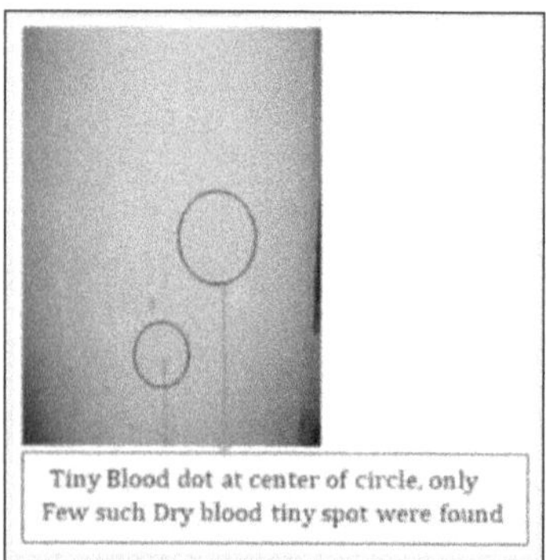

Figure 2 After collection of Scrapping

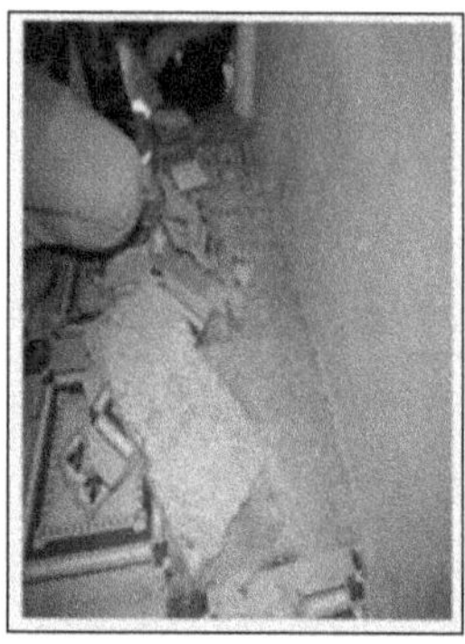

Figure 3 Floor was Dig to Verify the Blood

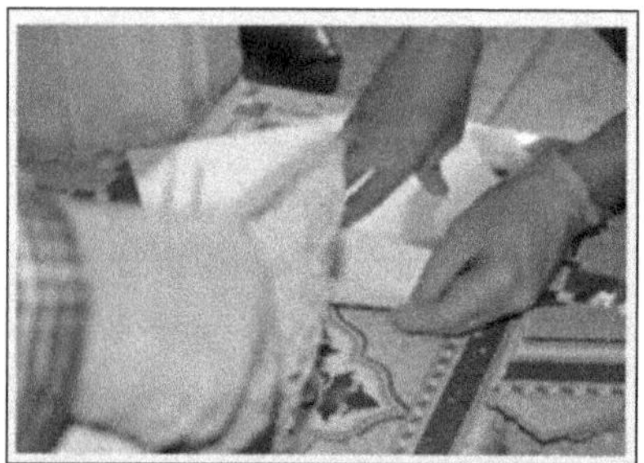

Figure 4 Collection of Scrapping on Paper

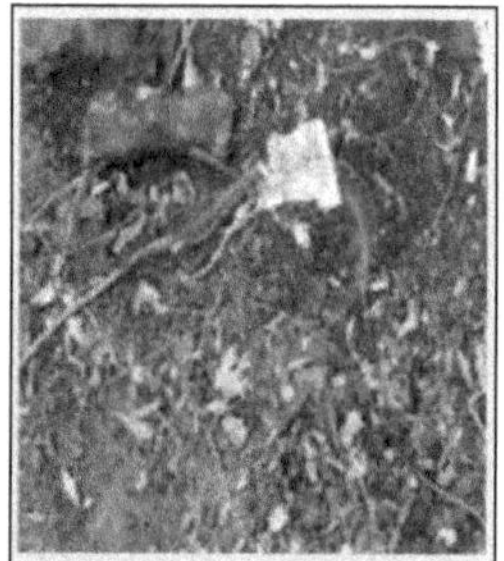

Figure 5 Traces of Burnt Tyre

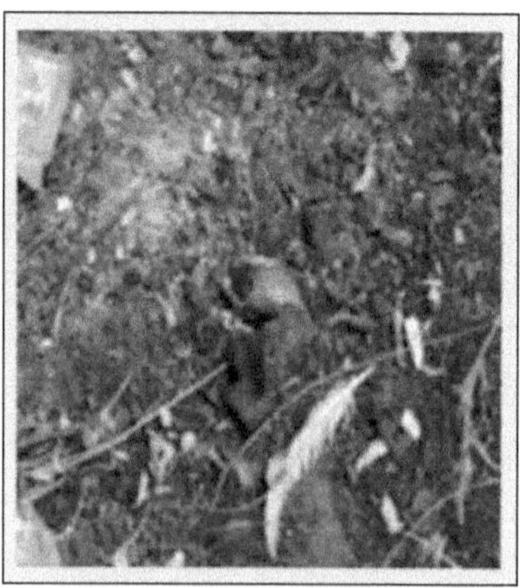

Figure 6 Traces of Burnt Tyre

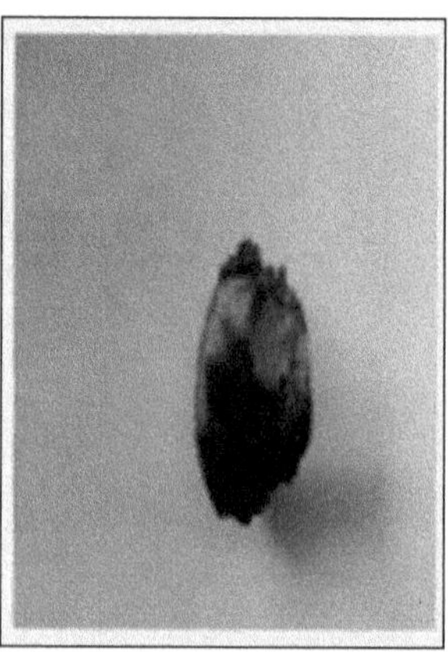

Figure 7 Partly burnt bone pieces found just few meters away from Neem tree

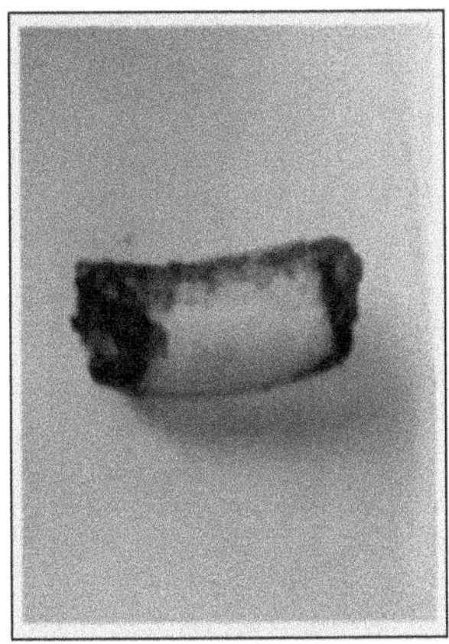

Figure 8 Partly burnt bone pieces found just few meters away from Neem tree

CONCLUSION

Even if the robbers make every attempt to erase evidence from the crime scene, scientific and appropriate monitoring of the location might always uncover some clues. One essential aspect of forensic skill is the meticulous collection of these hints. If there is a large amount of blood at the crime scene, swabbing can be useful; but, if there are little, dried drops of blood, scraping is recommended. That incident occurred twenty-four days prior, but fragments and partially burnt bones from the crime scene produced enough DNA profiles. These profiles were compared to his parents' and his identification was established. When DNA testing contributed to the case's resolution, the authorities were able to file a murder accusation.

SOURCES & REFERENCES

- https://images.app.goo.gl/gtH22TqRuHaVjwXz7
- https://medwinpublishers.com/IJFSC/IJFSC16000196.pdf

Chapter 2

MOCK MURDER IN 1996

Janu Reena J and Mohanapriya S

ABSTRACT

"Ragging does not break the ice, it breaks life."

Any disorderly behaviour that involves teasing, treating, or rudely handling any student, engaging in boisterous or indisciplined activities that create, or are likely to cause annoyance, difficulty, or psychological harm is known as ragging. This behaviour can be expressed verbally or in writing. Murder of a young man who studied in Rajah Muthiah Medical College, Annamalai University in Chidambaram, Tamil Nadu, India. Mr. Pon Navarasu, who was brutally murdered due to ragging. This incident led to the passing of the first prohibition of ragging act in Tamil Nadu in 1997.

INTRODUCTION

In the year 1996, a fresher named Mr. Pon Navarasu who was ragged and murdered by his senior Mr. John David. On 6th November, his body parts were crumbled and scattered into different parts of Tamil Nadu. His father, Mr. Ponnusamy, was a former vice-chancellor and a professor at Madras University. He filed a formal missing complaint on November 10th since Mr. Pon Navarasu did not turn up for Diwali celebration at his house in Chennai. After filing the charge sheet, the officer began the interrogation.

THE CASE

Scattered body parts

On November 7th, 1996, at Mandeville police station, Chennai, a police officer received a call from the conductor, Mr. Prakash, regarding a suitcase on bus route no. 21G from PTC bus depot at Mandaveli with a foul smell. Things happened quickly as the police unlocked the suitcase only to find male body parts scattered into pieces without a head, hand, or leg. The Chennai police officers then filed an FIR to initiate the investigation.

A MISSING CASE

On November 10th, 1996, a case was filed at Annamalai police station, Cuddalore, by a father named Mr. Ponnusamy that his 17-year-old son, Mr. Pon Navarasu, was missing. The police suspected that there might be a link between the suitcase present on the bus and the missing 17-year-old Mr. Pon Navarasu.

ON THE COMPLAINT LETTER

Mr. Pon Navarasu from Chennai continued his higher education by staying in a hostel. On November 6th, 1996, he called his father, Mr. Ponnusamy, to inform him that this was his last examination and after which he would be returning home for the upcoming Diwali celebration. On the 7th of November 1996, Mr. Ponnusamy grew anxious as his son did not turn up for the celebration. Another day passed for Mr. Ponnusamy to find out about the whereabouts of his beloved son. He contacted the college hostel only to discover that his son's room door was locked from the outside, indicating that he had already left. The hostel officials were not cautious enough as they assumed that Mr. Pon Navarasu was off for his Diwali vacation. After getting a clearer picture, Mr. Ponnusamy guessed that there might be a problem for his son on the way back home.

HOSTEL ROOM

Mr. Ponnusamy went to Mr. Pon Navarasu's college and informed them about the missing case of his son. They opened hostel room no. 95 of Malligai Hostel of Mr. Pon Navarasu and were shocked when they noticed that Mr. Pon Navarasu had not left the hostel for vacation as his belongings remained in his hostel room. The police started to investigate Mr. Pon Navarasu in the college, and during the investigation, they found out about his senior, Mr. John David, of the same college. Further investigations revealed that on November 6th in the afternoon, John had taken Mr. Pon Navarasu with him to his room.

THE HIDDEN SECRET

On November 11, Mr. John David surrendered in front of Mr. Raja Mannargudi magistrate by saying that he killed his junior. On November 18, police took Mr. John David into their custody. They started to investigate about Mr. Pon Navarasu, but he did not utter a word. In the midnight at 2.00 am, he started to gradually reveal some information. Mr. John David said that it was common for him to rag the first-year students. Since Mr. Pon Navarasu refused to follow Mr. John's instructions, which eventually led John's friends to disregard him, this greatly offended Mr. John. On November 6th, there was a match between India and South Africa, so every student in the hostel gathered in front of the television. As soon as Mr. Pon Navarasu completed his exam and returned to the hostel, Mr. John David blocked his way and took him to room 319 of KRM hostel, where he ragged him, made him naked, and forced him to lick and clean the shoe. When Mr. Pon Navarasu did not comply, he got triggered and took a metal rod, beating him on the head until Mr. Pon Navarasu fainted. Thinking he had died, Mr. John wrapped his head in a polythene cover, placing his chain, ring, and watch inside, then threw the cover in the dustbin behind his college. He then wrapped the body, leg, and hand in separate polythene covers, packed them in a suitcase, and boarded a Chennai train. On the way, he disposed of the hand and leg in a river, while he left the packed head with the suitcase on a town bus in Chennai before returning to Chidambaram out of fear. He surrendered to the police, providing this information, as stated by Mr. John David. Upon receiving this statement, the police changed the missing person report to a murder case. Following Mr. John David's information, the police searched the Annamalai college surroundings, checked the dustbin, and found Mr. Pon Navarasu's head. They also discovered a leg part near Chengalpattu. After examining these parts alongside the body tissue found in the town bus, they concluded that they belonged to Mr. Pon Navarasu.

Murder occurs due to ragging, creating fear among the people. The Tamil Nadu Government gives special attention to this case. On September 1, 1997, a charge sheet was filed in the Cuddalore session court. On the court's side, a special prosecutor named Mr.

Kandasamy, former Judge and defence lawyer Mr. Virudhachalam Reddiar, and Judge Mr. Singaravelu were involved. In the Cuddalore session court, the accused/respondent was found guilty under sections 302, 201, 364, and 342 IPC. He was convicted and sentenced to undergo life imprisonment under sections 302 and 364 IPC, rigorous imprisonment for one year under Section 342 IPC, and rigorous imprisonment for seven years. He was also ordered to pay a fine of one lakh rupees and in default to undergo rigorous imprisonment for twenty-one months under Section 201 IPC. A special act was enacted against ragging known as the "Tamil Nadu Prohibition of Ragging Act 1997", which defines ragging as the 'display of noisy, disorderly conduct, doing any act that causes or is likely to cause physical or psychological harm, or raises apprehension, fear, shame, or embarrassment to a student in any educational institution. It includes teasing, any type of physical injuries, or emotional injuries. Whoever directly or indirectly commits, participates in, abets, or propagates "ragging" within or without any educational institution shall be punished with imprisonment for a term that may extend to two years and shall also be liable to a fine that may extend to ten thousand rupees.'

As the trial process continued, there were seventy-eight witnesses, and 120 documents submitted. On March 11, 1998, the judgement given was double imprisonment for ragging and for hiding the evidence, and he was sent to Cuddalore central prison. This case did not close and proceeded to Chennai High Court in 2001. The judgement provided that the crime was not proved, and Mr. John David was set free. Tamil Nadu government took steps to prove the crime done by Mr. John David and appealed in Delhi Supreme Court against the decision made by the High Court to reopen the case.

APPEAL AGAINST ACQUITTAL

After ten years, the trial proceeded in 2011 on behalf of the Judge Mr. Dalveer Bhandari and Mr. Mukundakam Sharma. They provided the judgement as per the session court and evidence of circumstantial facts such as a shirt found on the terrace of KRM hostel and evidence such as fingerprints found on the polythene cover. The prosecution successfully established its case through compelling circumstantial evidence, and given the facts presented, it is impossible to find any alternative reasonable explanation that would support the accused. The High Court's perspective is completely incorrect and the result of improperly reading and analysing the available material. Given the discussion, facts, and circumstances of the case mentioned above, we believe that the High Court erred in overturning the trial court's finding of conviction because the prosecution had presented its case. As a result, we reverse the High Court's ruling and order and reinstate the trial court's ruling and decision.

IMPORTANT PICTURES FROM THE CASE

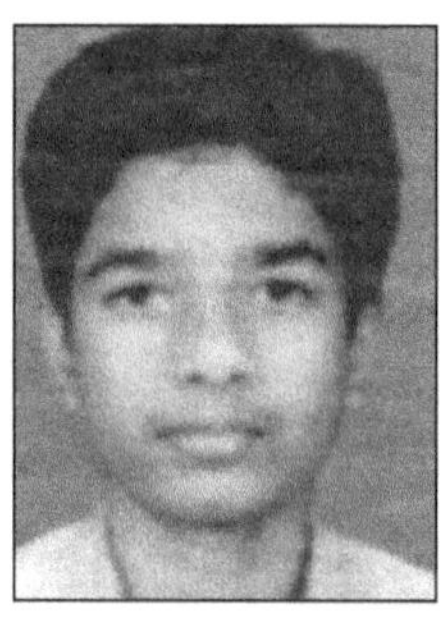

PON NAVARASU

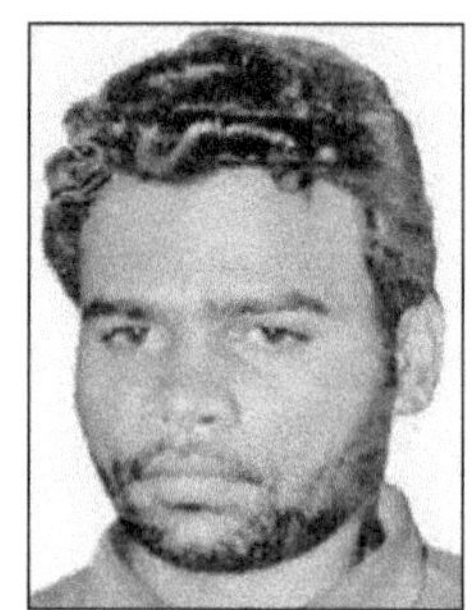

JOHN DAVID

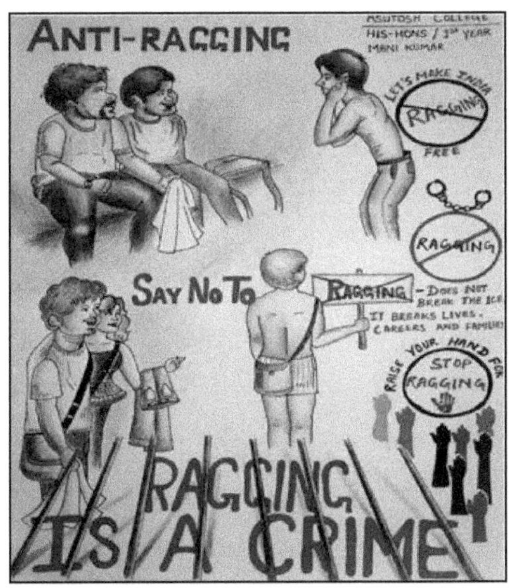

CONCLUSION

Say "no" to ragging. One person being killed by another without a valid reason or excuse under the law is intimidating a student to complete their work or keeping them from participating in university events. The legislation forbids certain types of bullying of kids, such as psychological distress and physical mistreatment.

FUTURE PERSPECTIVES

Dial the anti-ragging helpline number 0422-261-4324, 9487846635, 9487846549. Anti-ragging actions in the future are probably going to take a multifaceted strategy. Tougher laws and stricter enforcement will discourage would be offenders. To promote an inclusive and respectful society, educational institutions will place a strong emphasis on awareness and sensitisation campaigns. With the deployment of digital awareness campaigns, anonymous reporting platforms, and surveillance systems, technology will be crucial. Peer-led campaigns will encourage a sense of community and accountability by enabling classmates to actively oppose ragging. In order to address underlying difficulties, mental health support and counselling services will be essential. Peer mentorship initiatives and inclusive teaching methods will help incoming students transfer more smoothly. Evidence-based policies will be informed by research and data collection, and anti-ragging initiatives will be strengthened through cooperation with law enforcement and non-governmental organisations.

SOURCES & REFERENCES

- https://thefederal.com/states/south/tamil-nadu/navarasu-murder-in-1996-and-its-eerie-resemblance-to-shraddha-case/
- https://www.thehindu.com/news/national/revisiting-two-cases-of-medico-deaths/article66562792.ece
- https://timesofindia.indiatimes.com/city/chennai/david-the-killer-worked-in-city-b po-co-workers/articleshow/8068440.cms
- http://ponnaavarasutrust.org/evolution.html

Chapter 3

THE STONEMAN MURDERS

Gowtham T, Vinith Kiruba John Raj, AJ, and Kota Madhan Gopal

ABSTRACT

A serial murderer known as "The Stone Man" killed at least thirteen homeless persons in 1989 while they were sleeping in Calcutta. Between 1985 and 1988, a comparable string of killings in Mumbai was also attributed to the Stoneman. The murders are still unsolved and have never been connected to one another. According to Mr. Gupta, 60% of the plot in the film is fiction and 40% is truth. The murders are portrayed in the film as a police officer carrying out a religious ritual, and the mystery surrounding the murderer's identity persists. Director Mr. Srijit Mukherjee's Bengali film Baishe Srabon was released in 2011. The same enigmatic series of murders that occurred in Kolkata in 1989 served as the basis for the film's narrative. The murderer is shown in the film to typically target members of the underprivileged and destitute communities, such as street people, drug addicts, or sex workers. A glaring departure from reality occurs at the end of the movie when the serial murderer shoots himself after admitting to all of his atrocities.

Based on these events, producer Bobby Bedi created the movie the Stoneman Murders. At least thirteen homeless individuals in Calcutta were killed by the unnamed serial murderer known as "the Stoneman" in 1989. Following the sixth murder, the Mumbai Police identified a pattern in the crimes. A film titled "The Stoneman Murders" was made based on these incidents, but it deviates from the actual facts.

KEYWORDS

Stoneman, Mumbai, murder, homeless persons, 1989

INTRODUCTION
Mumbai Killings

1985. It was a calm and frigid night. Upper middle-class families were resting on comfortable mattresses draped with silky sheets. However, not everyone had the same privilege. A homeless guy slept in one of Mumbai's numerous dark alleyways. He could be thinking, "How will I feed myself tomorrow?" before going to bed. Unbeknownst to him, the first victim of 'the Stoneman' would die the next day. There is little information known about the individual other than that he was homeless and had no relatives. The victim's head was smashed by a stone weighing 30 kg. According to the plan, the Stoneman would select an unsuspecting victim sleeping alone in a deserted region and smash their head with a single stone weighing 30 kg. In most cases, the victims' names could not be determined since they slept alone and had no family or acquaintances to identify them. Most of the victims were homeless, and the crimes were not high-profile. It was not until the sixth murder that Mumbai police took the homicides seriously and noticed a pattern. The authorities assumed that the killer was a tall and well-built guy because the stones weighed up to 30 kg.

There was no motive, no proof, and no contemporary technology like CCTV cameras to help the police in their investigation. A homeless waiter escaped one of the Stoneman's assaults and managed to flee to report it to the police, but in the poorly lit part of Sion where he was resting, he could not get a decent glimpse of his attacker. Mumbai police tried everything to find the killer, including night patrols and apprehending persons who matched the murderer's description, but nothing succeeded. The killings came to an end in 1988. Mumbai could breathe a sigh of relief, but have the serial murders ended?

SUMMER OF 1989 IN CALCUTTA

The stone killings began in Kolkata in 1989, much to everyone's consternation. In reality, the Stoneman was a serial killer on the move. The first casualty was a lady who earned a living selling moonshine on the street; she died of head injuries. His second victim, a homeless beggar, was slain precisely one month later on July 4th. The Stoneman committed eleven additional killings. All of the killings followed a similar pattern: they were committed in a certain region (downtown Kolkata), all of the victims were homeless, and they were killed by having their skulls smashed with a 30kg stone. When police officers were sent around the city, they made several arrests. The killings stopped after a period of arrests, during which a limited number of "suspicious persons" were detained for questioning. However, the suspects were released into the public view owing to a lack of evidence. The crimes are yet to be solved.

GUWAHATI STONEMAN

After 20 years, six victims were murdered in 2009, following the exact same pattern as the Stoneman crimes, indicating that Kolkata police's beliefs regarding the Stoneman were incorrect. This instance is unknown, with only one paper available. It is as if this instance was not deliberately brought to public attention. This investigation was promptly concluded, with no one arrested.

FILM ADAPTATIONS BASED ON REAL-LIFE INCIDENTS

The Stoneman Murders, produced by Bobby Bedi, is based on real occurrences. The film was written and directed by Mr. Manish Gupta and stars Kay Kay Menon and Mr. Arbaaz Khan. It was released on February 13, 2009. Mr. Gupta says that his story for the film is 40% genuine and 60% fiction. The deaths are shown in the film as part of a religious ritual conducted by a police officer, with the identity of the true perpetrator left open to interpretation at the end.

THE STONE MAN KILLING

- The story began in 1989 in Mumbai's streets, with a terrifying atmosphere throughout the night.
- The tragedy was caused by an unknown masked ragpicker, according to police investigations.
- After six killings, detectives identified the killer's pattern.
- The suspect used a 30kg stone as a weapon and smashed the victims' heads with it.

MODUS OPERANDI

- The suspect targeted an unidentified victim sleeping alone in the streets at night.
- Police assumed the case involved unidentified bodies and cremated the body within 48-78 hours under IPC SEC 3.

- Because the victim was homeless, there were no relatives or witnesses to investigate the case.

SURVIVORS

- No proof or witnesses have been found thus far.
- The majority of the targets were killed, with only one survivor escaping to Calcutta.
- The event occurred as the waiter was coming home from work and preparing to sleep.
- The suspect attempted to hit the victim with a stone but fled with minor injuries on his head.

JOURNEY OF THE MURDER

- It began in 1985 on the streets of Mumbai.
- Within two years, 26 homeless people were murdered in Sion and Kings Circle.
- The violence spread to Calcutta in 1989.
- Calcutta police conducted a thorough investigation using various techniques.
- The murders were halted abruptly in mid-1988 due to a splatter and a split investigation.
- The pattern of killings was discovered in Guwahati in 2009.
- Desperate search and research.
- The pattern of murders perplexed Mumbai police.
- The suspect, which might be a single individual or many organisations, has yet to be identified.
- Comparable assaults occurred in Mumbai, Calcutta, and Guwahati, with comparable instruments, targets, and timing.

- Police departments encountered several conflicts.

- Evidence and eyewitness testimony was used to reach conclusions.

- Physical description: tall, well-built male.

- Police gathered information from many witnesses.

SUSPECTS

- Mr. Ramavat (2022)

- Mr. Shivprasad Dhruva (2022)

TRAIL (RAJKOT COURT 2016)

- In 2016, Mr. Hitesh Ramavat was arrested for stoning three persons.

- The Rajkot court acquitted him of two of the killings. The trial for the third murder is still underway.

Mr. Ramavat, 32, was acquitted by Additional Session Judge PN Dave of murdering tea seller Mr. Sagar Mewada and autorickshaw driver Mr. Ravin Barad. They shared a habit of sleeping on the street at night. The case is held in remand for 14 days due to insufficient evidence, with the benefit of the doubt applied.

SUSPECT (MR. RAMAVATH)

The apprehended was from Bedeshwar area of Jamnagar. He used to dwell in leased housing and usually stole his victims' cell phones. After taking the mobiles, he used to insert a SIM card to make calls to the banks requesting an ATM pin change. In 2016, Rajkot police deployed around 1,200 officers divided into squads to apprehend Mr. Ramavath.

EVIDENCES

- The prosecution has provided documentary evidence for the following.

- Recovered large stones from his leased property in Jamnagar, where he practised stoning.

- Victims' lost mobile phones were retrieved.

- Voice recordings of the suspect's interactions with bank personnel are presented in court as evidence.

CONCLUSION

The final verdict of these stone men was a mystery and an unsolved case; after a year of these killings, no clues, evidence, or eyewitnesses were discovered. Some claim that only one individual was responsible for these deaths, while others claim that a gang of people is to blame for this horrific event. Approximately half of Mumbai's 17 million inhabitants are homeless. Many were determined as suspects and detained, but owing to a lack of proof, all the crimes remained unresolved, and this individual is still a mystery today.

SOURCES & REFERENCES

- "8 Indian Serial Killers Who Will Give You GooseBumps". *IndiaTimes. 20 November 2014.* Retrieved 22 March 2021.

- ^ "The Stoneman Murders". *Criminal.* Retrieved 22 March 2021.

- ^ *Ghosh, Ritujay (30 December 2006).* "The elusive stoneman of Kolkata". *HinduSan Stimes.com. Ritujay Ghosh.* Retrieved 11 October 2018.

- Murder reported in 2004 similar to "Stoneman" killings of 1989. Report on alleged suspect in section of Times of India article from Jan 2004.

Chapter 4

A CASE STUDY OF A SERIAL KILLER: THE NOTORIOUS MR.TED BUNDY

Dharanidharan S, Aldrin Jebez E, Deventhiran M, Tholkappian E, and Arjun P

ABSTRACT

This case study explores the life and crimes of one of America's most infamous serial killers, Mr. Ted Bundy. From his childhood to his capture, trial, and eventual execution, the study delves into the twisted psyche of a man who murdered numerous young women and left a legacy of fear and fascination. Mr. Bundy's criminal activities, the investigation into his crimes, and the psychology behind his actions are examined in detail.

KEYWORDS

Mr. Ted Bundy, Serial killer, Theodore Robert Cowell, Criminal psychology

INTRODUCTION

Mr. Ted Bundy, born Theodore Robert Cowell, is an infamous serial killer in American history, known for his gruesome crimes, extensive criminal activities, and his ability to maintain a facade of charm and normalcy while committing heinous acts. This comprehensive case study delves into the life, crimes, and psychological intricacies of Mr. Ted Bundy, offering a deeper understanding of his reign of terror.

EARLY LIFE AND BACKGROUND

Mr. Ted Bundy's early life was marked by a web of family secrets, confusion, and a sense of abandonment. Raised to believe his grandparents were his parents and his mother was his sister, Mr. Bundy grew up with a distorted family dynamic. He excelled academically and in sports but carried the stigma of illegitimacy, possibly contributing to the development of his psychological disposition.

CRIMINAL BEGINNINGS

Mr. Bundy's criminal activities began in 1974 when he initiated a spree of abductions, rapes, and murders, primarily in Washington. His choice of victims, typically young women, and the gruesome nature of his crimes sent shockwaves through society. Mr. Bundy's intelligence, education, and charismatic demeanour allowed him to evade suspicion, making him a perplexing and enigmatic criminal.

INVESTIGATION AND ARREST

The investigation into Mr. Bundy's crimes was a complex and challenging process due to the absence of direct connections between him and his victims. However, persistent and diligent law enforcement efforts eventually led to him becoming the prime suspect. His initial arrest stemmed from a minor traffic violation in Utah, which ultimately led to his capture. Subsequent investigations unveiled Mr. Bundy's dark history and his connection to multiple unsolved murders.

PSYCHOPATHOLOGY

Psychological evaluations conducted during Mr. Bundy's time in custody raised red flags and suggested psychopathic tendencies. His manipulative and violent behaviour, evident even in his childhood, offered insight into the mind of a deeply disturbed individual capable of extreme cruelty. His psychological condition led to the origins of his violent tendencies.

LEGAL BATTLES

Mr. Ted Bundy's legal proceedings were marked by dramatic twists, including two successful escapes from custody. His intelligence and ability to represent himself in court allowed him to exploit legal loopholes, resulting in a complex and convoluted legal saga. These legal battles added to the mystique surrounding Mr. Bundy and further complicated his case.

CONVICTION AND SENTENCING

Mr. Bundy was eventually convicted of multiple murders, receiving sentences that ranged from life imprisonment to the death penalty. His confessions and the evidence presented in court left no doubt that he was a serial killer. However, the full extent of his crimes remains unknown, hauntingly leaving a legacy of unsolved cases.

LAST INTERVIEW

In his final interview before his execution on January 24, 1989, Mr. Bundy discussed his motivations and the lack of control he had over his murderous impulses. He attributed his violent behaviour, in part, to his troubled childhood and exposure to domestic violence. This interview provides a unique window into the psyche of a serial killer and the factors that may have contributed to his actions.

LEGACY

The Mr. Ted Bundy case continues to have a profound impact on the field of criminal psychology and the public's perception of serial killers. Mr. Bundy's ability to seamlessly blend into society while committing heinous crimes serves as a chilling reminder of the dangers posed by individuals with psychopathic traits. The case has sparked extensive academic and public interest, leading to further research and discussions on criminal psychology and the intricacies of serial killers.

CONCLUSION

The case of Mr. Ted Bundy stands as a chilling example of the depths to which human depravity can sink. His capacity to elude capture, manipulate the legal system, and maintain a facade of normalcy while committing a series of gruesome murders makes him a unique and unsettling figure in criminal history. Mr. Ted Bundy's legacy extends beyond his crimes, leaving a lasting impact on the way society views and studies serial killers.

SOURCES & REFERENCES

- https://www.britannica.com/biography/Ted-Mr.Bundy
- https://en.m.wikipedia.org/wiki/Ted_Bundy

UNRAVELLING MYSTERIES WITH FORENSIC ENTOMOLOGY: A CASE STUDY IN AN INSECT-ASSISTED INVESTIGATION

Amirthabashini N, Dheebashri S, and Sania Mirza C

ABSTRACT

Forensic entomology involves the study of how insects and arthropods can be applied to criminal investigations. The life cycles of insects serve as accurate timekeepers in this sector, beginning soon after death. The study of insect life cycles becomes essential in determining the post-mortem interval (PMI) when other techniques are unable to offer the required information. Forensic experts can determine the length of time since death, any shifts in the corpse's location, and even the reason for death by observing the insect population and the stages of larval development.

This book focuses on the distinctive qualities of the regional insect fauna observed on human corpses in two places, Al-Manfuha district of southern Riyadh and Florida. It explores the dynamics of these insects' interactions with human remains and how they can help with forensics to solve the cases. During autopsies, the insects were removed from human corpses. The study's main goal was to collect necrophagous insects that live on human remains and learn more about how they might help with criminal investigations.

KEYWORDS

Forensic entomology; Post-mortem interval (PMI); Insect colonisers; Larval development; Necrophagous insects

INTRODUCTION

Insects and other arthropods can be used as evidence in court proceedings, according to the discipline of forensic entomology. It necessitates an in-depth comprehension of insect taxonomy, ecology, physiology, and biology in relation to legal issues. In addition, the insects found at crime scenes in particular geographical areas are crucial in answering the fundamental concerns of violent crimes, such as where, when, and how the victim was involved in the incident. By seeing the succession of arthropods on the deceased body and comprehending their developmental stages, the time of a person's death can be inferred. The post-mortem interval (PMI), the mobility of the corpse, the manner and cause of death, and probable connections to suspects at the crime scene are all understood through the use of insect colonisers. Many different kinds of arthropods view a decomposing corpse as a valuable food source.

Insights can be gained from researching insects discovered on or nearby cadavers. In death investigations, especially when dealing with extensively decomposed or skeletonised human remains, accurate study and interpretation of insect evidence are very crucial. Insects and humans are often regarded as the most successful organisms on Earth. Blowflies are the first to arrive at a body, followed by beetles and other insects. The sorts of insects present and their developmental stages can be used to determine when a death happened. Insect-related evidence can provide vital details on drug use, child and elder abuse, sexual assault, the hiding or moving of a body after death, victim identification, the location of injuries sustained prior to death, and post-mortem alterations to a body and its surroundings. The ultimate objective of any criminal investigation is to establish a solid link between a suspect and the scene of the crime or a suspect and a victim. In order to be considered as reliable, evidence relating to insects should be given the same importance as other sorts of evidence such as bloodstains, fingerprints, hairs, fibres, or any biological elements. Recent studies have highlighted the critical importance of following the right methods while gathering and conserving entomological evidence. Such evidence, when properly acquired, can also offer insightful information for revisiting unsolved cases and presenting crucial evidence in court. In the ever-evolving subject of forensic entomology, case reports are essential because they demonstrate the field's usefulness in real-world situations. The field has a long history of using classic case studies to demonstrate the efficacy of forensic entomology. A good place to start was Dr Kenneth G.V Smith's 1986 book, which had nineteen prominent examples. Following this, scientists all across the world conducted in-depth studies, such as the 1991 work by Mr. Goff and Mr. Flynn, who calculated post-mortem intervals (PMI) by examining the patterns of arthropod succession in a number of case studies.Here we present two human cases in Riyadh, Florida, highlighting the type of insect evidence used, considering the impact of habitat and the stage of decomposition.

THE CASES
CASE 1
Detailed Description

The crime scenario that is being described is fictitious, yet it is reminiscent of a number of actual forensic entomology incidents in which insects were essential in identifying the offender. In this case, Ms. Pamela Martin, a 55-year-old lady, was found dead on Mount Cabin, Florida, on March 30th, in a very decomposed state. Mr. John, her spouse, discovered her corpse while strolling down a trail that led to their shared mountain cabin. On March 1st, the Martins had travelled to their cabin. Mr. John was required to leave shortly after, leaving Ms. Pamela alone as he went to work in the northeastern region of the state. Former school librarian Ms. Pamela Martin had spent her retirement years reading and caring for her garden. She lived a quiet, modest existence, taking medication for her arthritis and heart disease. Mr. John had been married to Ms. Pamela for thirty years, but he was frequently gone for significant amounts of time due to his work as a long-haul truck driver. The pair did not have any kids. The closest neighbours were many kilometres distant from their cabin, which was situated in a remote area. There was no internet connection, and the cell phone reception was spotty. Despite these difficulties, the couple continued to make frequent trips to the cabin; on occasion, Mr. John would leave Ms. Pamela alone to complete his trucking routes throughout the state.

INVESTIGATION

The police and coroner showed up at the spot on March 30, the day after Mr. John reported Ms. Pamela's body via his Citizen Band radio. The team of forensic entomologists gathered entomological evidence as the police interviewed John and his neighbours to record their testimonies.

SUSPECT INTERVIEWS

Ms. Pamela's husband, Mr. John Martin, had worked in low-wage sales positions in the past and was concerned about losing his truck driving job. Three months before, it was discovered that he had taken out a $500,000 life insurance policy on Ms. Pamela, which made him the main suspect in the case.

The general store owner, Ms. Julia Snow, had lived in the area for her entire life and knew a lot about the local gossip, which made her stay ten km away from Martin's cottage. After the couple's March 1ˢᵗ visit to the store, Julia told the police she had not seen Ms. Pamela Martin. The closest neighbour, Ms. Ashley Bright, who lives in the next cabin five km away, used to work at the local store when she was a teenager. But it was believed that she was now dependent on small-time thefts and drug dealings to support herself. Ms. Ashley stated that she had only seen Ms. Pamela the previous year and that she had only seen the Martins a few times, although she did say that Ms. Julia had informed her of the Martins' March 1ˢᵗ trip to the cabin. If Ms. Pamela Martin indeed died on March 1ˢᵗ when she arrived at the cabin with Mr. John, then Mr. John becomes the primary suspect. By examining the species and life stages of insects discovered in and around the body, forensic entomology can determine the exact time of death. Ms. Pamela Martin's body was at the decaying stage when it was found on March 30, thus the insect involved in this investigation process was Phaenicia sericata (Fig. 1).

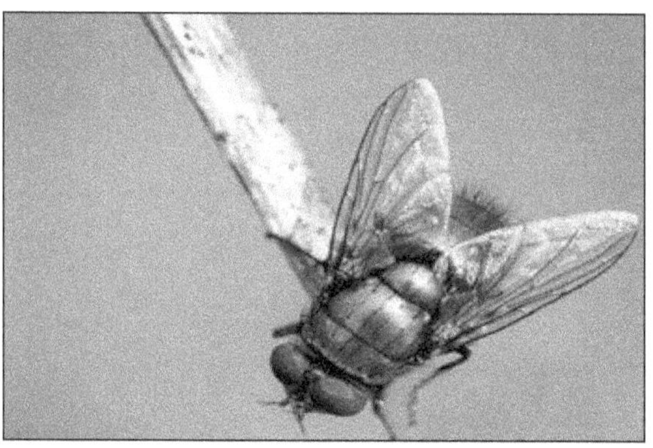

CASE 2

Detailed Description

An adult male's lifeless body **(Fig. 2)** was found in a partially enclosed flat in the Al-Manfuha district in the southern portion of Riyadh on March 7, 2017. The victim was discovered in a room with partially open windows. The body lay on the ground, dressed in bulky springtime attire with long sleeves, sport pants, and briefs underneath. The observed level of decomposition was late bloated stage, as evidenced by a strong stench, substantial abdominal distension, and prominent facial and neck swelling along with protrusion of the tongue and eyes.

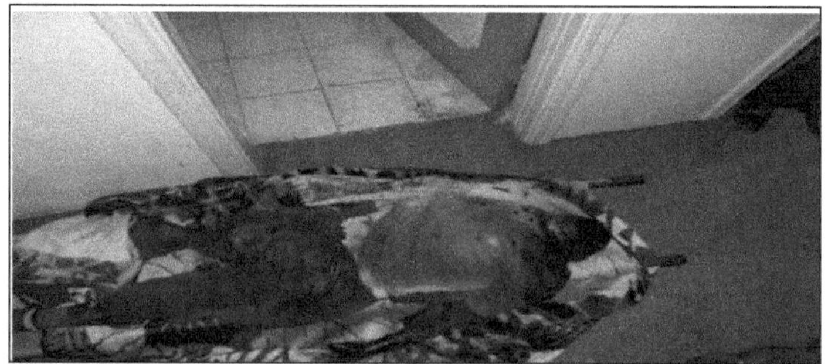

INVESTIGATION

The police inquiry revealed that the last verified sighting of the person was four days prior to the corpse being found. In the week preceding the body's discovery, the local weather station closest to the scene of death registered an average temperature of 27.5 ± 1.7 °C.

During the course of the inquiry, crime scene investigators discovered seven different stages of insect life on the deceased person's clothing. There were two larvae, two pupae, and three adults among them. The samples that were gathered were then sent to King Saud University's Entomological Laboratory for additional analysis. The specimens were identified using a reference key, and it was concluded that they belonged to the second stage of the decomposition process, Musca domestica (Fig. 3).

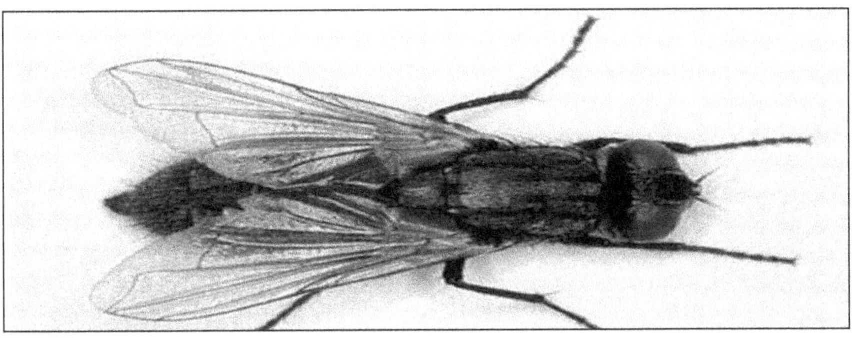

Based on the entomological data and the pathologist's findings, four days were determined to be the estimated post-mortem interval (PMI).

DISCUSSION OF THE CASES, RELATED TO FORENSIC ENTOMOLOGY

Before going into the discussion, first, we have to know about forensic entomology.

When it comes to pinpointing a more exact time frame for killings, forensic entomology is crucial. In order to identify possible suspects, verify alibis, and acquire a thorough grasp of the circumstances surrounding the murders, detectives need this information. It also offers important proof that can be used in court to help prosecute criminal cases.

To put it simply, forensic entomology analyses insects found in and around crime scenes to help determine the time of death. Attracted to decaying bodies, insects follow a recognisable colonisation and succession cycle. Forensic entomologists can provide information about the length of time the bodies have been dead by looking at the kinds of insects, their life cycles, and their developmental schedules. The ability to narrow down the potential time periods that the crimes might have occurred depends on this information. There are normally five phases of decomposition, and temperature and environmental factors can affect how quickly these stages change.

The stages of degradation or decomposition and the corresponding insects are as follows:

1. Fresh Stage: This phase begins at the moment of death and ends when bloating starts.

2. Bloated Stage: The body fills with gases that are released by bacteria during this stage.

3. Decay Stage: As decomposers pierce the skin, gases escape. Fly maggots (including Calliphoridae and Sarcophagidae) and other Diptera species, such as little dung flies, army flies, scuttle flies, and black scavenger flies, become active and begin feeding on the corpse.

4. Post Decay Stage: At this stage, bone, cartilage, and skin are all that is left.

5. Skeletal Stage: At this point, all that is left are bones and hair.

NOW COMING TO THE CASES

In Case 1

Clusters of adult maggots were collected by the forensic entomology team from the victim's mouth, nose, and abdominal wound, which the coroner subsequently determined was caused by a 20 × 4cm knife blade. These maggots, which belonged to the blow fly species **Phaenicia sericata**, were primarily in the late third stage of decomposition. This species pupates after around 10 days, at an average temperature of 20°C, which is common in the area during March, according to the nearby weather station. No pupae or pupal cases were found around the body, even after a thorough search, which was to be expected if the maggots had been active from March 1st to the 19th. Considering this data, we concluded that Ms. Pamela's death could not have happened any sooner than March 20th.

As no one had seen Ms. Pamela alive since they arrived at the cabin together on March 1st, Mr. John Martin was suspected of having a motive. Nevertheless, evidence from forensic entomology suggested Ms. Pamela was present until at least March 20th. It raised doubts regarding John's whereabouts on that occasion if he was the offender. However, since Ms. Pamela Martin frequently shopped at Ms. Julia Snow's general store when visiting her cabin, it appears that Ms. Julia Snow had no desire to hurt Ms. Pamela Martin. Julia remembered that Ms. Ashley Bright had come into the store sometime around March 20th, looking dishevelled and with what seemed to be bloodstains on her shirt. In response, the police obtained a search order for

Ms. Ashley's cabin, where they found Ms. Pamela Martin's empty prescription vials. Furthermore, Martin's kitchen knife was recovered from the septic tank and matched the description of the murder weapon. The widely held belief was that Ms. Pamela had challenged Ms. Ashley while she was attempting to take her vital prescriptions, which led to a fatal confrontation in which Ms. Pamela was stabbed with her own knife while attempting to get her medications back.

Due to the timeframe provided by forensic entomology, which showed that Ms. Pamela could not have been killed before March 20th, the police ultimately named Ms. Ashley as the main suspect in Ms. Pamela's slaying. The fact that Ms. Ashley was at Ms. Pamela's cabin at that time and that her shirt was covered in blood were important factors in this decision.

In Case 2

The information provided by the Forensic Entomologists:

1. Decomposition Stage: The corpse was in the bloated stage of decomposition. This stage typically follows the initial stages of decomposition, such as the fresh and active decay stages.

2. Age of the Decedent: The age of the individual in this case was 40 years.

3. Clothing: At the time of discovery, the corpse was clothed. This can be relevant for understanding the circumstances surrounding the death.

4. Manner of Death: The manner of death in this case was determined to be natural death. This suggests that the cause of death was due to natural causes rather than external factors like homicide or accident.

5. Location: This was an indoor case, which means that the corpse was found indoors, and the conditions for decomposition were influenced by the indoor environment.

6. Reporting and Documentation: The case was reported and documented in March, which could be important for establishing a timeline and understanding the environmental conditions at the time of discovery.

7. Insect Samples: Twelve dead insect samples were collected as part of the forensic investigation. These samples included three adults, seven larvae, and two pupae. All the specimens collected belonged to the species Musca domestica L., which is commonly known as the housefly.

8. Insect Activity: The presence of houseflies in the semi-closed indoor case suggests that they were attracted to the decomposing body. Insects like houseflies are often used in forensic entomology to estimate the post-mortem interval or time since death based on their life cycle stages and the environmental conditions.

9. Developmental Data: The development of Musca domestica larvae was studied, and it was noted that at a temperature of 27.5°C, it took four days for the larvae to reach the third instar.

10. Post-Mortem Interval (PMI): The estimated post-mortem interval (time since death) was determined to be 4 days based on both the pathologist's report and police investigation, considering the last time the deceased was seen.

11. Agreement between Forensic Pathology and Entomological Data: The PMI derived from the entomological data (insect evidence) aligned with the PMI estimation based on forensic pathology.

This information, which describes the decomposition stage, entomological evidence, and other pertinent elements in establishing the time of death in a particular case, seems to be a part of a forensic investigation report. Forensic specialists should take into account many pieces of evidence, including entomological data, in order to arrive at a more precise estimation of the post-mortem interval.

This information provides an overview of the forensic inquiry into the natural death of a forty-year-old man in an indoor environment, highlighting the role of housefly activity and presence in determining the post-mortem period.

TABLES

The most relevant data concerning human cases and the insects that have infested them, including the number of insects and their life stages (adults (A), larvae (L), and pupae (P)) should be considered.

CASE NO	AGE (YEARS)	GENDER	DECAY STAGE	AMBIENT	SCENE	COLONIZED INSECTS	FINDING MONTH	PMI ESTIMATION
1	55	FEMALE	DECAYING	INDOOR	CAMR. BIN	PHANAECIA SERICATA	MARCH 1ST	5 DAYS
2	40	MALE	BLOATED	INDOOR	SEMI-CLOSED APARTMENT	MUSCA DOMESTICA	MARCH 17	4 DAYS

CONCLUSION

The forensic examination into both deaths, based on the material presented, mostly relied on entomological evidence to establish important details regarding the date and circumstances of death. In each case, initial doubts about the manner and timing of death were confirmed or disproved in large part by the meticulous study of insect activity and developmental phases. This emphasises how important forensic entomology is in offering insightful information for criminal investigations. In this instance, forensic entomology was able to provide an important timeframe for the death, which helped to reduce the range of possible times when the death might have happened.

In a nutshell, forensic entomology is an indispensable instrument in criminal investigations, particularly when determining the exact moment of death. In all situations, determining the post-mortem period and locating possible suspects were greatly aided by bug evidence. In order to establish their cases and guarantee that justice is done, law enforcement and the legal system need this information.

SOURCES & REFERENCES

- Gennard D.E. John Wiley & Sons; Chichester, England: 2007. Forensic Entomology: An Introduction.

- Hall R.D. Perceptions and status of forensic entomology. In: Byrd J.H., Castner J.L., editors. *Forensic entomology-The utility of arthropods in legal investigations.* CRC Press; Boca Raton: 2001. pp. 1–16.

- Hall, R.D., 2008. Forensic Entomology. In: Capinera, J.L. (Eds.), Encyclopedia of Entomology. Springer Netherlands, pp. 4346.

- Introna F., Campobasso C.P., Di F.A. Three case studies in forensic entomology from southern Italy. *J. Forensic Sci.* 1998;43:210–214.

- Sukontason K, Narongchai P, Kanchai C, Vichairat K, Sribanditmongkol P, Bhoopat T, et al. Forensic entomology cases in Thailand: a review of cases from 2000 to 2006. *Parasitol Res.* 2007;101:1417–23.

- Smith K.G.V. A manual of forensic entomology. London: Trustees of the. *British Museum (Natural History)* 1986

- Kreitlow KLT (2009) Insect succession in a natural environment, In: Byrd JH, Castner JL (eds.), Forensic entomology: The utility of arthropods in legal investigations, (2nd edn). Boca Rotan, FL: CRC Press, USA, pp. 251- 269

- Amendt J., Richards C.S., Campobasso C.P., Zehner R., Hall M.J.R. Forensic entomology: Applications and limitations. *Forensic Sci. Med.*

- *Pathol.* 2011;7:379–392. doi: 10.1007/s12024-010-9209-2.

- Campobasso C.P., Introna F. The forensic entomologist in the context of the forensic pathologist's role. *Forensic Sci. Int.* 2001;120:132–139. doi: 10.1016/S0379-0738(01)00425-X.

- Amendt J., Anderson G., Campobasso C.P., Dadour I., Gaudry E., Hall M.J.R., Moretti T.C., Sukontason K.L., Villet M.H. Standard Practices. In: Tomblerin J.K., Benbow M.E., editors. *Forensic Entomology—International Dimensions and Frontiers.* Taylor & Francis Group; Florence, KY, USA: 2015. pp. 381–398.

- Bugelli V., Campobasso C.P., Verhoff M.A., Amendt J. Effects of different storage and measuring methods on larval length values for the blow flies (Diptera: Calliphoridae) *Lucilia sericata* and *Calliphora vicina. Sci.Justice.* 2017;57:159–164. doi: 10.1016/j. scijus.2016.10.008.

- Bugelli V., Campobasso C.P., Zehner R., Amendt J. How should living entomological samples be stored? *Int. J. Leg. Med.* 2019;133:1985–1994. doi: 10.1007/s00414-019-02114-0.

- Magni P.A., Harvey M.L., Saravo L., Dadour I.R. Entomological evidence: Lessons to be learnt from a cold case review. *Forensic Sci. Int.* 2012;223:e31–e34. doi: 10.1016/j.forsciint.2012.09.001.

- Smith K.G.V. A manual of forensic entomology. London: Trustees of the. *British Museum (Natural History)* 1986

- solving-crimes-by-using-forensic-entomology https://ww1. odu.edu/content/dam/odu/offices/reyes/docs/reyes-week-2-presentations / solving-crimes-by-using-forensic-entomology

Chapter 6

ARIYALUR GANG RAPE CASE 2016

Viswalakshmy V. M., Madhumitha S., and Esther Beula M.

ABSTRACT

Sexual abuse is a common and a serious public health problem in our society. We present a case of a pregnant Dalit woman who was brutally raped by four upper-class men. Their intention was to kill the baby. Her vagina was cut with a blade, and the fetus was pulled out of her womb. We highlight a case of rape that happened in the district of Ariyalur, Tamil Nadu.

INTRODUCTION

This case is all about a 17-year-old pregnant Dalit girl named Ms. Nandhini who was gang-raped by a Hindu Munnani Union Secretary and three of his friends in December 2016 in Ariyalur district. Police reports revealed that the Hindu Munnani Union Secretary was irked at Ms. Nandhini, insisting on marrying her after she got pregnant by him after being in a relationship with him.

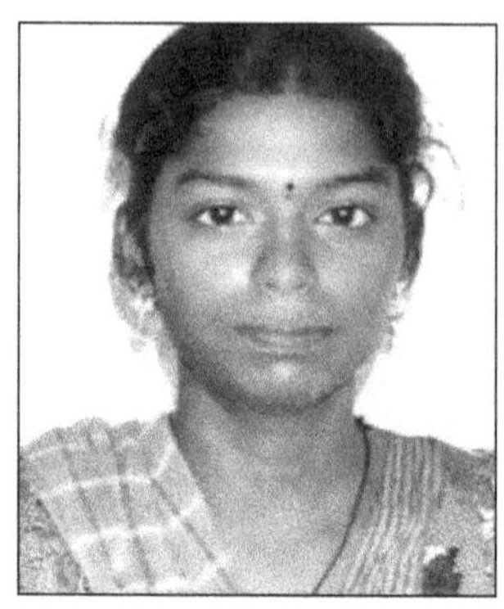

THE CASE

Ms. Nandhini, daughter of Mr. RAJENDRAN and Mr. RAJAKILI, belonged to the Sirukadambur village in Ariyalur district. She is from a Dalit community. She has an elder brother and elder sister. After the death of her father, she could not continue her studies after 8th std. After that, she started helping her family with construction work. She fell in love with Mr. Manikandan [aged 26] belonging to the dominant caste Vanniyar community [HINDU MUNNANI UNION SECRETARY], who was also a worker on the same construction site. After being in a relationship for more than a year, she got pregnant. After this incident, she compelled Mr. Manikandan to marry her, but he refused to marry her because of caste issues. He was also pressuring her to abort the fetus, but she was completely against it.

The case goes like this: on 29 December 2016, Ms. Nandhini went missing. The family members went on searching for her. On the same day at 8.30 pm, Ms. Nandhini's mother's relative named Ms. Venila received a call from Ms. Nandhini, and she said that she was in love with a person named Tamilarasan in VELLUR. On that day, Ms. Nandhini's mother filed a kidnapping case and mentioned that she had doubts about Mr. Manikandan. On 30 December 2016, the family again filed a kidnapping complaint against Mr. Manikandan, mentioning that he had kidnapped their daughter, but the police insisted they change the kidnapping case to a missing case. Thus, the police proceeded with a missing complaint.

[SEC 361]

This is in breach of Section 361 of the Indian Penal Code, which explicitly specifies that if a minor is taken away without any of the proper permission of their guardian, the child is kidnapped. The police registered the FIR on 5th January 2017 and began an enquiry. Devi, a close friend of Ms. Nandhini, was questioned by the police and she informed the police about the relationship between Ms. Nandhini and Mr. Manikandan and about pregnancy matters. Mr. Manikandan was called for an enquiry on 5th January by Irumbulikurichi police. But on behalf of the signed witness, he was allowed to go. Due to Mr. Manikandan's significant political connections, the police allegedly showed bias in his favour, and he subsequently went into hiding the following day. On 9 January 2017, police started questioning the friends of Mr. Manikandan. On 12 January 2017, Mr. Manikandan was admitted to the hospital; he committed suicide by consuming poison in the village of Kodukkur. The Kuvaagam police station filed a case and took Mr. Manikandan's confession. He confessed that he committed suicide because of being caught for the murder of Ms. Nandhini.

After the police investigations on the Hindu Munnani Union Secretary, they found Ms. Nandhini's body on 14 January. The police confessed that she was abducted by Mr. Manikandan. Three days later, she was gang raped. Later, they cut her genitalia with a blade and pulled out the fetus from her womb. Their main intention was to kill the baby. Due to excessive bleeding, Ms. Nandhini was pronounced dead. They tied her hands and then tied her body with a stone and threw it into a well. To avoid further complications, they killed a dog and put its body in the same well. The partly decomposed body of Ms. Nandhini was found in the village of Sirukadambur. She was found with her hands tied at her back and her clothes and jewellery stripped off.

On 14th January, Mr. Manikandan surrendered to the village administrative officer and confessed his crime. Mr. Manikandan was arrested under the Goondas Act and was jailed at Trichy central prison. Mr. Manikandan's friends were arrested on 15th January 2017. The family believes that one more person has also been involved in the crime. According to the family, the Hindu Munnani district secretary is also a part of the crime because he works with Mr. Manikandan. The Ariyalur police reported that there is proof against the district secretary, while Mr. Sasikumar proclaimed that the Hindu Munnani district secretary had not been enquired at all.

AUTOPSY

The autopsy results revealed that Ms. Nandhini was gang raped. On the basis of the post-mortem examination, it is revealed the level of body decay. The police confessed that her death happened two weeks before the body was discovered. The victim's family was not satisfied with the reports. Advocate Sasikumar claimed that Ms. Nandhini had been seen with Mr. Manikandan till 3rd January. The family claimed that the police were attempting to fix the death date as 29th December in order to cover up the inability to find out the victim.

POLICE TREATMENT

Ms. Nandhini's family was ill-treated by police officials. Ms. Nandhini's mother said that the DSP had visited their home on 16th January and mocked them. Her mother also stated that she had never seen her daughter in an improper way.

COURT VERDICT

On April 2017, the High Court of Madras ordered Criminal Investigation Department [CB-CID] to investigate the crime. Justice Mr. R. Mahadevan gave the directive after seeing Ms. Nandhini's mother's original complaint. In April 2019, the Madras High Court declined to transfer the rape case to CB-CID. Justice GK Ilanthiriyan ordered the police to apply sec 376 D of IPC to the charges and to conclude the inquiry within 6 months.

CONCLUSION

In this case, Mr. Manikandan was not punished because of a lack of proper evidence. In conclusion, I would like to convey that sexual violence poses an obstacle to the peace and security of women in society. Many women have lost their health, studies, family, etc., as a result of rape. Similar to the Ariyalur case, there are millions of cases which remain unsolved. Punishments should be made more severe to stop sexual offences in our society.

SOURCES & REFERENCES

- https://en.wikipedia.org/wiki/2016_Ariyalur_gang_rape_case#Backg round
- https://www.deccanchronicle.com/nation/current-affairs/060217/was-ariyalur-girl-gang-raped-killed.html

Chapter 7

THE MS. ENO FARIHAH CASE

Arul Darshini A, Jothi S B, and Sakthisri S

ABSTRACT

tIn Tangerang, Indonesia, on the night of May 14, 2016, 19-year-old Ms. Eno Farihah invited her new boyfriend Mr. Rahmat Alim (age 16), whom she had been dating for a month. In her home, Mr. Rahmat tried to get Ms. Eno to have sex with him, but she rejected his advances. Mr. Rahmat was furious and left sulking. He returned a few hours later with two other men, Mr. Bin Hartono (age 24) and Mr. Imam Harpiadi (age 24). They forced their way into Ms. Eno's home and pushed her to the ground. One of the men covered her face with a pillow while the other went looking for a knife, but all he could find was a dining fork and a garden hoe that were nearby. The two 24-year-old men raped her, cut her face with the fork, and smothered her until she was unconscious. Mr. Rahmat refused to rape her because the bleeding from her face disturbed him, so instead, he bit her on the breasts and legs. One of the men then inserted the handle of the garden hoe inside Ms. Eno's vagina and kicked the blade as hard as he could. The hoe impaled her up to 60 cm deep, rupturing most of her internal organs, including her lungs. They then covered her body with pillows and blankets before fleeing. Three days later, Ms. Eno's body was discovered by two of her work friends who went to her home to check on her after they grew worried when she had not turned up for work. Mr. Rahmat, Mr. Bin, and Mr. Imam were easily tracked down and arrested a few days later. Mr. Bin and Mr. Imam got the death penalty, but it is not sure if it has been carried out yet or if they appealed. Mr. Rahmat was sentenced to ten years' imprisonment.

KEY WORDS

1. **INTERNET:** A global computer network providing a variety of information and communication facilities, consisting of interconnected networks using standardised communication protocols.

2. **MEME:** An image, video, piece of text, etc., typically humorous in nature that is copied and spread rapidly by internet users, often with slight variations.

3. **SEXUAL VIOLENCE:** Someone forces or manipulates someone else into unwanted sexual activity without their consent.

4. **RAPE:** To force someone to have sex when they are unwilling, using violence or threatening behaviour.

INTRODUCTION

May 15, 2016, Indonesia. A 19-year-old girl named Ms. Eno Farihah was living in a district called Tangerang in Indonesia. This girl was working in a plastic factory there, and she did not come to the office for three consecutive days. Her friends got suspicious and thought that Ms. Farihah might be sick. So, they called and texted her, but there was no reply from Ms. Farihah, and the call was left unanswered. Ms. Farihah was not someone who disappears without anyone's notice.

When they went to investigate Ms. Farihah's room, the door was locked. They knocked on the door, but there was no reply. They got suspicious, broke the door, and entered the room. As soon as they entered the room, they sensed a horribly rotting smell. When they looked around the room, Ms. Farihah was not there. In the corner of the room, over the bed, a lot of clothes were piled up. The scene they saw when they moved the clothes was an unforgettable tragic scene in their life. Ms. Farihah was naked, her face was destroyed, a hoe was inserted completely into her private part, and she was lying dead. A very gruesome crime scene. A woman should always feel safe; even a little negligence will turn a safe situation into a brutal and extremely dangerous one. Awareness measures must be taken to avoid these situations in the future. So, what happened to Ms. Eno Farihah? Who killed her so cruelly? Did the police find them or not?

THE CASE

The 19-year-old Ms. Eno Farihah completed her degree, and she was working in a plastic factory. There is accommodation to stay and work near the factory, and it is separate for men and women. Ms. Farihah's house was a little far from the company, and hence she decided to stay in company-provided accommodation. Even during her work times, she visits her home often. Ms. Farihah's parents had seven children, and Ms. Farihah is the fourth child. Ms. Farihah's parents decided to get her married exactly a month from now, that is in April 2016.

Who is Mr. Rahmat?

A 16-year-old boy named Mr. Rahmat came and started talking to her. While talking like that, both of them exchanged their phone numbers and subsequently started conversing on their phones every day, which eventually led them into a relationship. Since Mr. Rahmat is only 16 years old, he was studying in junior school. His school was a short distance from the place where Ms. Farihah was staying. At the same time, Ms. Farihah's family did not know about this untold relationship between them. When Ms. Farihah came to know that her parents were looking for a groom for her marriage, she requested Mr. Rahmat to end their relationship as she would not go against the decision taken by her parents whatsoever. Mr. Rahmat agreed to that, with the strong condition that she should gift him with a kiss before ending their short-term relationship. On 12 May 2016, Ms. Farihah told Mr. Rahmat to come to the room where she was staying.

What really happened that night?

The time was exactly 11:30 at night, and it was raining heavily outside. Ms. Farihah invited Mr. Rahmat into her room. The design of the room was such that there were many separate rooms in a compound with a separate section for both men and women. There was even a big gate between these two sections which always remained locked. Ms. Farihah and Mr. Rahmat were alone in the room as everyone had separate rooms in the compound. Both were talking for a while, and Ms. Farihah explained her situation to make him understand. Nevertheless, at one point, as Mr. Rahmat insisted, they were involved in kissing each other.

While kissing, Mr. Rahmat started undressing Ms. Farihah. As Ms. Farihah understood that it was going beyond a kiss, right away, she stopped by saying she was not interested in having sex with him, which led to complications for her and her family as her marriage was also fixed. So, she asked Mr. Rahmat to leave. This sexual rejection of Ms. Farihah made Mr. Rahmat feel very shameful and he left the room angrily. He went out and stood in an area between the girls' room and the boys' room and started smoking a cigarette. That is when two unknown guys approached him.

About the criminals

The guys who were staying in the men's dormitory, a 24-year-old Mr. Hartono and Mr. Imam Harpiadi working in the same plastic factory, came over there and started enquiring about Mr. Rahmat. He was explaining the love relationship with Ms. Farihah, and it had come to an end too. All three of them started talking for a while and came to know about each other. At one point, both asked Mr. Rahmat to take them to his girlfriend's room. They all started moving slowly towards Ms. Farihah's room and stood in front of the room, then slowly started turning the door handle of Ms. Farihah's room. However, to their surprise, the door was unlocked as Ms. Farihah went to sleep without locking her door.

"This is a common mistake that many people make, since they think that it is safe to stay in their room or at home. Who might come there and will be careless, but if the time is not right, even a normal situation will change into a very dangerous situation."

All three of them opened the door and went inside the room and saw Ms. Farihah sleeping in her nightdress. Soon both Mr. Imam and Mr. Hartono recognised that this Ms. Farihah was the one who was working with them. Mr. Imam was working in the same department at the same factory where Ms. Farihah works. Earlier, Mr. Imam had shown keen interest in Ms. Farihah and tried several crooked ways to contact her, which was unsuccessful, and Mr. Hartono knows about this very well.

CRIME SCENE

As Mr. Hartono was thinking about the humiliation undergone by Ms. Farihah due to his ugly-looking face and body, the three of them were looking at Ms. Farihah who was sleeping there. Immediately, Mr. Imam took a pillow from the side and pressed it into Ms. Farihah's face, and soon Ms. Farihah awakened. Without knowing what was happening to her, she started moving her hands and legs in order to escape. Instantly, Mr. Imam took a fork from the side and started punching Ms. Farihah's face rapidly. At the same time, Mr. Hartono grabbed her arms and legs to stop her from moving. Then both of them called Mr. Rahmat, who was looking at them, and asked him to bring a knife from somewhere. Right away, Mr. Rahmat also searched for a knife everywhere, but the knife was nowhere to be found. So, he came out of the room and started looking for where to find a knife.

While searching for a weapon, he got a sight of a garden hoe. He quickly grabbed it and went into Ms. Farihah's room. He saw Ms. Farihah's face was covered in blood, and he forcefully hit the iron part of the hoe on her face as ordered by Mr. Imam. This made Farihah lose consciousness. Without even an ounce of guilt, Mr. Imam and Mr. Hartano raped Ms. Farihah. However, Mr. Rahmat refused to do so as the blood-covered face of Ms. Farihah disturbed him. Instead, he crazily bit Ms. Farihah's chest, leg, and thigh. Mr. Hartono took that hoe and inserted it into Ms. Farihah's private part. Since it did not go inside further, he kicked with his legs and pushed deeper inside heavily. Until then, Ms. Farihah was alive, but soon after this barbaric act, it damaged the internal organs, and she died in a few minutes. Now after killing Ms. Farihah, they washed all the blood stains on their bodies. After that, they stole some things from Ms. Farihah's room, including her mobile phone. Subsequently, they piled up all the cloths over Ms. Farihah, who was lying dead on the bed. They locked the room door from outside and fled away, leaving behind a lot of evidence.

ARRIVAL OF POLICE AT THE CRIME SCENE

Police came to the crime scene immediately, and Ms. Farihah's body was taken for autopsy. The cause of death was reported to be massive internal bleeding. The handle of the hoe was 60 cm inside Ms. Farihah's body and was kicked with terrible force. The handle of the hoe, which went in with high force, damaged Ms. Farihah's heart, lungs, and other organs severely.

Due to excessive loss of blood from the internal organs of Ms. Farihah, she died on the spot. Forensic experts collected as many pieces of evidence from Ms. Farihah's body, including saliva, fingerprints, bite marks, semen, etc. As soon as the news broke, all the other women who were staying in that factory accommodation room vacated immediately as they feared this brutal incident and their safety aspects. Instantly, the police started the investigation and began tracing Ms. Farihah's mobile phone. On the night of the incident, both Mr. Imam and Mr. Hartono were roaming around late at night, as the police came to know about it through the factory workers. The police personnel caught both, inquired, and searched their rooms only to find bloodstains on their clothes. After the analysis of the bloodstains, it was confirmed to be Ms. Farihah's blood. Subsequently, all three were arrested in the next few days, and an inquiry was conducted by the police.

Firstly, when Mr. Rahmat (Ms. Farihah's boyfriend) was inquired, he reasoned that Ms. Farihah was not ready to marry him since her parents had already been searching for a groom. She also denied the to proceed with the personal relationship with him, which eventually irked him. Secondly, Mr. Hartano was humiliated by Ms. Farihah, since she stated that he was unattractive. Lastly, Mr. Imam was being ignored by Ms. Farihah, which led him to commit this brutal rape and murder.

The DNA of the three accused was perfectly matched with the evidence collected. After that, the crime scene enacted by them was broadcast live on television.

THE COURT SCENE

In 2017, the case started in court and what happened to Ms. Farihah was explained in detail at the court along with the relevant evidence. When it was read in the court, Ms. Farihah's mother, who was present there, began to cry, as all the small details that happened to her daughter were read in the courtroom. Not only that, but she also saw the advocate who was present in support of the three murderers and asked him, "Do you have any conscience? They have killed my daughter so cruelly; how can you support them? Are there no girls in your house?"

If anything like this happened to the girls in your home, will you come and support them? she asked. In addition, she also asked "how you can sleep peacefully every night." However, there was no reply from that advocate.

PUNISHMENT FOR CRIMINALS

Finally, the court gave a death sentence to Mr. Imam and Mr. Hartono. Only 10 years' imprisonment was given to Mr. Rahmat as he was 16 years old at that time, though he was also proved to be guilty. This caused a lot of anger among the people. A lot of people started gathering in the court to take revenge on him. The police tried to stop them and, in the process, both sides clashed, and some officers were severely injured. When this case was already going very disturbingly, some people in Malaysia started laughing by creating memes on the horrible incident that happened to Ms. Farihah. Some of the pictures are below.

1. **The Criminals**

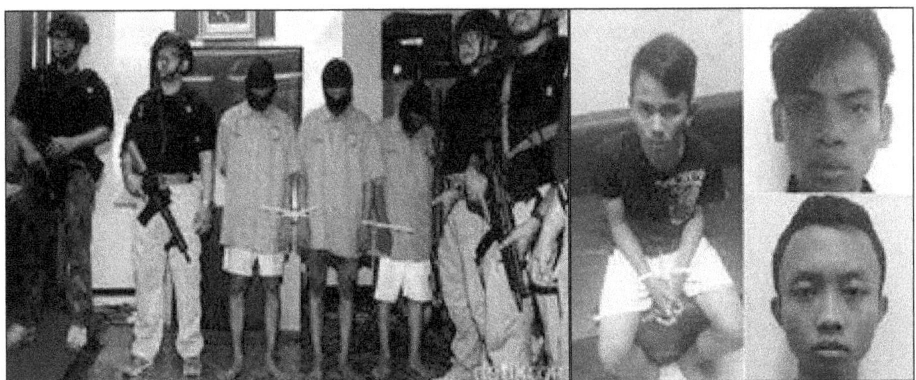

2. **The Weapon used**

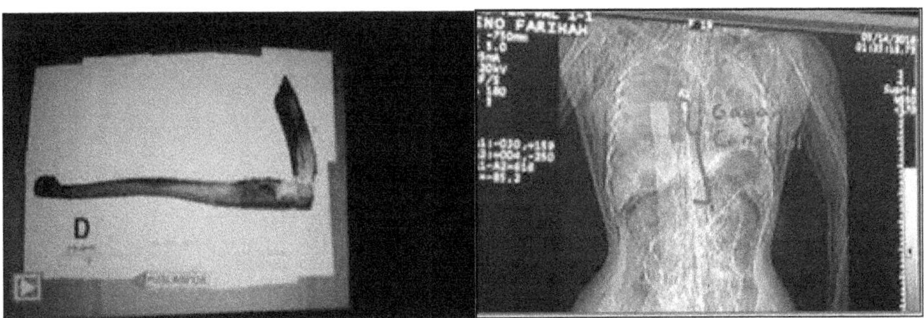

3. Ms. Eno, Mr. Ms., Ms. Farihah.

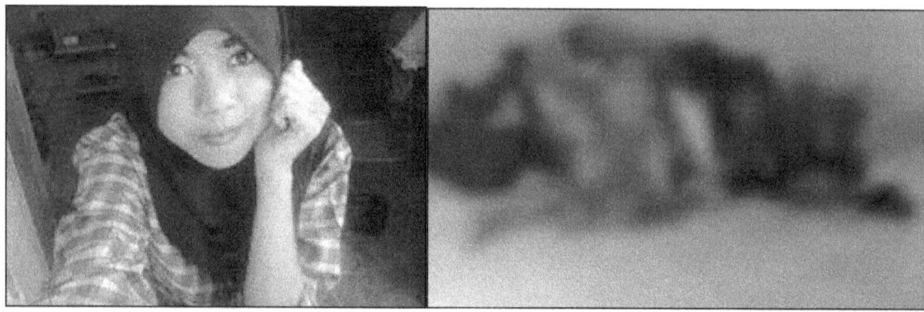

CONCLUSION & PERSPECTIVE

As we have gone through the series of crime scenes, we must always be conscious of what is happening around us. Always avoid meeting strangers in an isolated place and instead meet them in a public place. If her negligence of not locking the door and the carelessness had changed, she might have been alive today.

SOURCES & REFERENCES

- https://en.tempo.co/read/844429/Judge-hands-down-death-penalty-to-Ms. Eno-Mr. Ms. Ms. Farihah s-killers

- https://creepycuriosities.squarespace.com/the-murder-of-Ms. Eno-Mr. Ms. Ms. Farihah

- https://www.eyerys.com/articles/timeline/teenage-girl-raped-and-stuffed-hoe-and-how-people-memed-it-laughs?page=2#event-a-href-articles-timeline-alphabet-panicked-when-samsung-considers-replacing-google-with- Mr. Bingalphabet-039-panicked039-when-samsung-considers- replacing-google-with-Mr. Bing-55-billion-lost-in-market-value-a

Chapter 8

HATHRAS GANG RAPE AND MURDER

Aleen Godina A S and Geethan N

ABSTRACT

In September 2020, a nineteen-year-old woman belonging to a Dalit community was raped, but *via* investigation, it was alleged as a culpable homicide because of the caste which played a major influence in this case. Although the crime had happened and the victim was holding her last breath, the aftermath incident that happened to the dead body by the Uttar Pradesh police was a horrible incident for the victim's family. There were many turning points in this case which led to the judgement as culpable homicide. This case exposes the caste-based and gender-based discrimination which may be a systematic failure in the Indian criminal justice system.

KEY WORDS

Hathras - Gang Rape - Uttar Pradesh - Caste-Based Discrimination - Gender Discrimination - Victim's Rights - Marginalised Communities

INTRODUCTION

> **Unless we address the root "cause caste" and take into account the structures that enables caste atrocities and sexual violence against Dalit women, there is no way forward**

The Hathras gang rape case is a tragic incident that deeply exposes the grim reality of sexual violence, caste-based discrimination, and systematic injustice in India. The case involves the horrifying assault of a 19-year-old Dalit woman, which sparked public outrage and protests across the country. This case study is an example of irresponsible police investigation and misuse of power. The influence of the upper caste in the case makes the situation even worse.

THE CASE

The case date was not September 14, 2020; it started ten years ago. The rapist's family intentionally discriminated against the victim's family based on their caste. Once the victim filed a complaint against the grandfather of the rapist under the Prevention of Atrocities Act, 1989, which led to the arrest of the grandfather and enraged the family. On the date mentioned above, the victim and her mother went into the farm to collect cattle feed and dry sticks for cooking. The victim was a little far away, about 100 metres from her mother, searching for sticks. Sometime later, being partially deaf, her mother found only one of her foot leg slippers in the field. Seeing that, her mother got scared and started searching for her. Within ten minutes of searching, she found her daughter in a pathetic state, totally undressed near a tree, with her neck surrounded by her dupatta, and holding her last breath. The last word uttered by her daughter before her death was the name

"Mr. Sandeep," who happened to be the grandson of that family. Initially, she went to the police station and narrated the happenings and her daughter's condition. Hearing all this, the police filed the case as an attempted murder. She was admitted to the Jawaharlal Nehru Medical College and Hospital in Aligarh on 14 September, with her spinal cord severely damaged. She was later moved to the Safdarjung Hospital in Delhi after her condition worsened. Despite several treatments given, she died on 29 September 2020. Doctors reported that the cause of death (COD) was injury to the cervical spine by blunt-force trauma. However, according to her mother's statement, Mr. Sandeep Thakur and Mr. Luvkush Thakur harassed Miss Manisha Valmiki (the victim), leading to her daughter's death.

The UP police took the body from the Delhi hospital and brought it back to Hathras without the consent of the parents. The police cremated the dead body at 2.30 am as per the ADG (law and order) after obtaining consent from the family members, but this was not true. The news at first was considered fake news, and later a UP police officer reopened the case and stated that it was not rape as no sperm was found according to the forensic report. From the point of view of other experts, they said that a swab test for sperm should be performed if the rape occurred within the previous three days. If it is delayed, then a swab test should be taken for semen under the condition that not only the presence of sperm, but various other aspects also determine the probability of rape cases.

The UP government also hired a public relations firm and published a press release on behalf of the government stating, "the Hathras teenager was not raped."

INVESTIGATION

The case was then handed over to the CBI after the notification from the central government.

After the arrest, the accused Mr. Sandeep Thakur stated to the police that "I and Miss Manisha Valmiki were friends and regularly talked through phone calls, but her family was against our friendship and so we killed her." Accordingly, the UP police proceeded with the investigation and collected the call record details. In that around 100 calls were made from the phone which was registered in her brother's name between October 2019 and March 2020. Finally, the Hathras police arrested the four of them and charged a case under attempt to murder and gang rape. On 19 December 2020, CBI submitted the charge sheet to the court along with the charges. The CBI's final document reported that 115 calls were recorded between the victim and the accused.

JUDGEMENT

The court, in the judgement, released three of the four members involved (Mr. Ramu, Mr. Luvkush, and Mr. Ravi). However, Mr. Sandeep was convicted under the offences of culpable homicide not amounting to murder (IPC Section 304) and provisions under the SC/ST Act, but not for rape and murder. He was sentenced to life imprisonment along with a fine of ₹50,000.

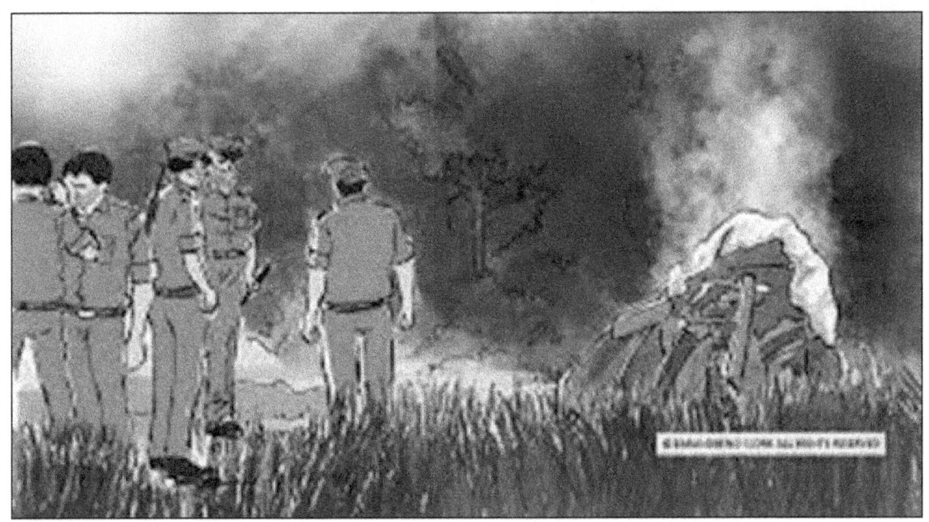

Nineteen-year-old Dalit woman was burnt by the police in
Uttar Pradesh's Hathras without the consent of her parents

CONCLUSION

In conclusion, it was seen that if you are born in a lower caste, you may be discriminated against by the upper caste. Seeking justice as a lower caste always remains a difficult task.

FUTURE PERSPECTIVE:

- The constitutional system and the judicial system should be strong in a way that these kinds of discriminatory assaults will be avoided.
- Providing basic awareness about Article 15 among society.
- Ensuring the protection and rights of these marginalised people.
- An overall solution is that "A CASTE-FREE SOCIETY."

SOURCES & REFERENCES

- https://en.wikipedia.org/wiki/2020_Hathras_gang_r   ape_and_murder

- https://www.thehindu.com/news/national/other-states/dalit-girl-gangraped-by-upper-caste-men-in-uttar-pradeshs-hathras-dies-in-delhi-hospital/article32721406.ece

- https://timesofindia.indiatimes.com/india/rape-survivor-moved-to-delhi- spine-damage-permanent/articleshow/78375589.cms

- https://www.thehindu.com/news/national/hathras-gang-rape-pposition-parties-demand-resignation-of-up-chief-minister-yogi-adityanath/article 32734523.ece

- https://mumbaimirror.indiatimes.com/opinion/columnists/pritish-nandy/another-girl-raped-and-   murdered/articleshow/78524751.cms

- https://www.bbc.com/news/world-asia-54351744

- https://www.hindustantimes.com/lucknow/hathras-   gangrape-accused-were-harassing-her-for-months- says-mother-of-19-year-old/story-6MwdIIiEG2x7KHN0BUkQDN.html

Chapter 9

THE BEST REAL-LIFE REVENGE OF ALL TIME

Lathika Sree V, Priya D, Harshini S, and Subhiqsha S

ABSTRACT

Mr. Bharat Kalicharan, infamously known as Mr. Akku Yadav, was a notorious Indian serial killer and rapist who terrorised the city of Nagpur, Maharashtra, in the late 1990s and early 2000s. His reign of terror ended in 2004 when he was lynched by a mob of over 200 women from the Kasturba Nagar slum, where he had committed many of his heinous crimes. Mr. Yadav's crimes included rape, murder, and extortion, with estimates suggesting he was also responsible for nineteen murders and numerous rapes. His case highlights the failures of the Indian criminal justice system and the need for community-driven action against serial offenders. This abstract provides a brief overview of Mr. Yadav's crimes and the circumstances surrounding his death, serving as a starting point for further exploration into the psychological, sociological, and criminological factors that contribute to such heinous behaviour.

KEYWORDS

Oppression, Mob Lynching, Revenge, Social classes, Gangsters, Molestation, Rape, Serial rapist, Extortion, Home invasion, Robbery, Kidnapping, Abduction, Political power, Police support, Vigilantism, Women Empowerment.

INTRODUCTION

Nemesis is a punishment or defeat that somebody deserves which cannot be avoided. Karma is viewed as a sum of a person's good and bad acts which affect their fate. Revenge is harm done to somebody as a punishment for harm that they have already done to someone, and there are several other sets of theories that describe getting paid back. Mob Lynching is an informal act done by an informal public group to punish any offender or a group. Mob lynching expresses an inferior sign of violating the law and is common in many countries like Kenya and South Africa. Mr. Bharat Kalicharan, notoriously known as Mr. Akku Yadav, was a serial killer and rapist who unleashed a reign of terror in the city of Nagpur, Maharashtra, India, during the late 1990s and early 2000s. His brutal crimes sent shockwaves throughout the community, leaving a trail of devastation and despair in his wake.

Mr. Yadav's exploits were marked by their sheer brutality and brazenness, with his victims primarily being women and children from the marginalised communities of Nagpur's slums. His crimes went unchecked for an alarmingly long period, exposing the systemic failures of the Indian criminal justice system and the societal apathy that allowed him to operate with impunity. However, in a dramatic turn of events, Mr. Yadav's reign of terror came to an end in 2004 when he was lynched by a mob of over 200 women from the Kasturba Nagar slum, who had been victimised by his heinous crimes. This incident sparked a national conversation about vigilantism, gender-based violence, and the need for community-driven action against serial offenders. This book delves into the life and crimes of Akku Mr. Yadav, examining the psychological, sociological, and criminological factors that contributed to his transformation into a monster. Through a nuanced exploration of his case, we aim to understand the complexities of serial offending, the failures of the justice system, and the resilience of the human spirit in the face of unimaginable horror.

THE CASE

The people of Kasturba Nagar, Nagpur, India, lived through a terrible period between 1991 and 2004. There lived a man named Mr. Bharat Kalicharan, also known as Mr. Akku Yadav, who accustomed himself to maltreat the people of a particular caste residing in the basti (slum). He was an extortionist, serial killer, home invader, and a gangster of the locality. He took control of almost 400 families in the basti for about 13 years.

It is filed in the police record that Mr. Akku has raped about forty women and Mr. Akku has been charged in twenty-six criminal cases. In most of the cases, he was taken into custody along with his gang members. Akku had a very suspicious nature; he doubted every outsider investigating about him. He would threaten people in case anyone complained about him. No women were safe in the locality; he always had a bad eye on women. Mr. Akku once, between 4:00 and 5:00 am, invaded a woman's house, stabbed and locked up her husband, and abducted the woman to somewhere, where she was raped for 4 hours. He would beat up even the poor old people if they failed to give him money. Ms. Maya, one of his victims, states that Mr. Akku stripped and burnt the inner thighs of her husband with a cigarette, sexually assaulted her, and made Ms. Maya dance for him in front of her young daughter.

Many houses in the basti had broken doors and broken roofs. The poor people pulled out their daughters from school and protected them behind the veil of zananas, so no one could see them. Almost twenty-five families migrated from the town to other places as they were not able to sustain such cruelty. Even casual conversations were restricted in the area for both men and women. He even prohibited children from playing together. He, along with his gang, raped girls as young as 10 years old, newlywed brides, and pregnant women to express his inhuman attitude. Mr. Akku had both police support and political power; he would bribe the policemen with the money he had snatched from the poor people.

The residents of Kasturba Nagar were left with only two possibilities:

- *Being puppets in the hands of Akku and bearing all his ferocity, or*

- *To join his gang and support him in his inhuman activities.*

For this reason, the people never built enough confidence to counterattack him.

He was settled as a sadist with his modus operandi being rape and control over 400 families in the locality. He realised the people's ideology in case of rape and molestation and accomplished his ideas to fulfil his needs. The bitter truth is everyone who was not in the play gets angry & expresses their indignation, and blames every middleman including government, politicians, chauvinists etc.

Besides everything, have you ever put yourself in the place of a victim of rape? Just picture yourself in it, what will be your next move?

Crying at the corner? Suicide? Blame Everyone? Or REVENGE?

Will you fight for your justice? Will you really explain everything to your family and folks to make them understand and stand alongside? A bit tangled case, right? Of course, it is not always as easy as criticising others. Raising a voice for one's own self has always been a more difficult task than raising voice for others.

People subjected to the burden of cruelty always wait for a hero to enter; they wait for a fearless, brave, and courageous character who could come and save them by performing the so-called heroic activities. The same ostensible idea applies in this case. Mr. Akku mapped out that to threaten or control someone, he must rape any woman in the family. The ideology is: in case he rapes any woman or girl in the family, the men in the family get embarrassed about the family's honour and obey him. The men of Kasturba Nagar have neither opposed nor fought against the rapist. But why? Why haven't they fought? Why did they leave some lunatic serial rapist to take control over them? Out of grief? Out of fear? Fear of what? Fear of the rapist carrying the word of what he did and confessing to everyone that he had raped the women of your family in a very proud and hearty manner. What in the world is even the point of the rapist feeling proud about? What makes a man feel so proud of himself in raping a woman?

Why does this social stigma always stigmatise the victims of rape and not the rapists?

Mr. Usha Narayane was a 22-year-old native resident of Kasturba Nagar and one of the few educated people in the locality. One day, as usual, when Mr. Akku threatened and intimidated a woman, Ms. Ratna Dungiri in her house, demanding money. Following this, Ms. Usha interrogated the scene and urged Mr. Dungiri to inform the police. When the poor frightened woman refused, Ms. Usha herself approached the police and filed a complaint, which later provoked Mr. Akku. The police illegitimately informed him about Ms. Usha's petition.

Enraged, Mr. Yadav marched to Ms. Usha Narayane's house with the gang of forty members. Ms. Usha shut herself inside the house and declined to confront the situation. The mob started invading her house. They also threatened her, saying she would be subjected to gang rape and acid attacks. However, this brave girl refused to surrender herself till the end and fearlessly frightened them back, threatening to burst the LPG cylinder in the house, which made Mr. Akku, and his gang run out of fright. This incident gave a lift to the oppressed people, and all of them now started gaining a positive spirit and became powerful enough with the confidence that emerged from Ms. Usha's bravery. Subsequently, people started attacking Mr. Akku by throwing stones at him and his peers. The people even set fire to Akku's house. Hence, he had no choice for survival in the basti, sought self-protection from the police station by surrendering himself.

When Mr. Akku was taken for a bail hearing on 13th August 2004 to the district court of Nagpur, an angered mob of more than a hundred men and women marched towards the court with weapons with the intention to attack Mr. Akku. When Mr. Akku was brought in by policemen, he walked in and verbally mocked one of his rape victims among the mob, saying that 'HE WOULD RAPE HER AGAIN AFTER RETURNING TO THE BASTI'. Right after that, he was attacked cruelly by the mob simultaneously. The woman he mocked told him, "WE BOTH TOGETHER CANNOT LIVE IN THIS WORLD; IT IS EITHER YOU OR ME".

Mr. Akku was subsequently lynched by a huge mob of hundreds of women inside the courtroom. The policemen who tried to save him were also attacked; women dusted chilli powder on the faces of policemen who tried to protect him. The angered mob kept stabbing Mr. Akku even after he was dead; his blood had splattered everywhere around the courtroom. As per the record, Mr. Akku's corpse had a count of at least seventy stabs. The police later arrested Ms. Usha Narayane and twenty-one others on charges of murder. A crowd of more than 500 people came forward to support Ms. Usha and demanded her bail by surrendering themselves for the act of lynching.

From torturing women to being killed at the hands of the same women is the ironic plot twist in the story of a man who lived as a brutal, sadistic, vicious serial rapist. After reading the whole story, aren't you already excited to see the man who existed to be such a menace to society? Look him up.

PICTORIAL REPRESENTATION

Before

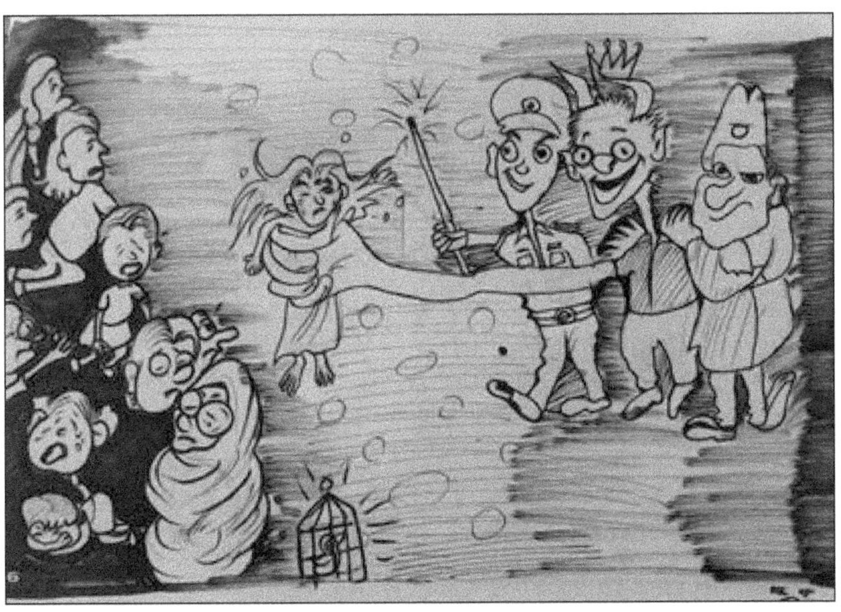

After

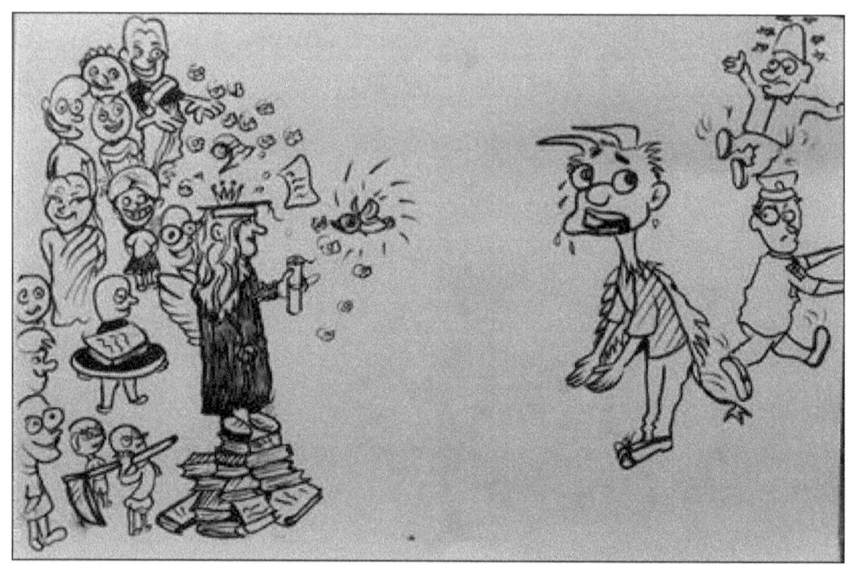

SOURCES & REFERENCES

- https://timesofindia.indiatimes.com/city/nagpur/Decade-after-Akkus-courtroom-murder-all-accused-go-free/articleshow/45104117.cms

- https://www.nytimes.com/2006/01/15/opinion/in-india-one-womans-stand-says-Ms. Enough.html

- https://humanrightsinitiative.org/publications/police/killing_justice_vigilantism_in_nagpur1.pdf

- https://www.theguardian.com/world/2005/sep/16/india.gender

- https://timesofindia.indiatimes.com/india/Women-proud-of-lynching-goon-in-court/articleshow/815580.cms

Chapter 10

2019 HYDERABAD GANG RAPE AND MURDER

Varsha. S, Theresa Pathrose and Harini. S

ABSRACT

The gang rape and murder of a 26-year-old veterinary doctor in Shamshabad, near Hyderabad, provoked outrage across India in November 2019. Her body was discovered on November 28, 2019, in Shadnagar, the day after she was murdered. Four individuals were apprehended and admitted to raping and killing the doctor, according to Hyderabad Metropolitan Police.

KEY WORDS

Gang Rape, Murder, Veterinary, lorry drivers, CCTV.

INTRODUCTION

Dr. Ms. Priyanka Reddy, a veterinary physician from Shamshabad in Hyderabad, was discovered lifeless along with her body partially burnt beneath Chatanpalli bridge in Shadnagar on Thursday morning. She had worked as a healthcare provider in Kolluru village. The incident occurred on Wednesday evening. She was raped, smothered, and then burnt by four men who were said to be hailing from Narayanpet.

On Friday, four people were apprehended by Hyderabad police. They had been identified as Mr. Mohammad Areef (driver), Mr. Jollu Naveen (cleaner), Mr. Chennakeshavulu (cleaner), and Mr. Jollu Shiva (driver). According to the police, the accused saw Ms. Priyanka parking her scooter at the Shamshabad toll plaza while drinking alcohol and devised a plot to rape her. One of them (Jollu Naveen) punctured the back wheel of the doctor's scooter, which was already parked.

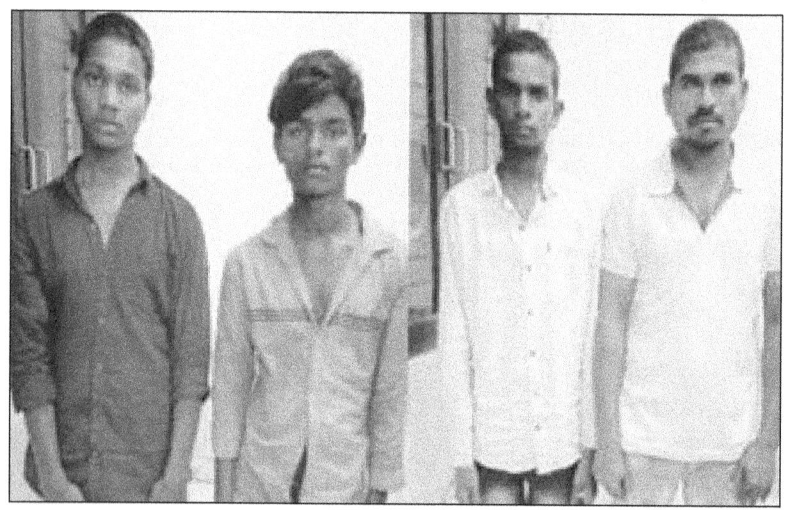

THE CASE

In November 2019, the gang rape and murder of a 26-year-old veterinary doctor in Shamshabad, near Hyderabad, sparked outrage across India. Her body was found in Shahnagar on 28th November 2019, the day after she was murdered. Four suspects were arrested and, according to the Hyderabad Metropolitan Police, confessed to having raped and killed the doctor. On 27th November 2019 at around 6:15 p.m., after parking the scooter, the victim took a taxi to a dermatologist's office in Hyderabad. The suspect parked her scooter near a toll plaza. After returning at around 9:15 p.m., she noticed the flat tyre and made a call to her sister. Two lorry drivers and their acquaintances noticed her. They deliberately let the air out of her scooter tyre, acted like they wanted to help her, and then forced her into nearby bushes. There, they sexually assaulted her and suffocated her. She continued screaming for help, so the men poured whisky into her mouth to silence her. When she regained consciousness, they smothered her, wrapped the corpse in a blanket, transported it in their truck 27 km to a location near the Shahnagar interchange on the Hyderabad Outer Ring Road, and at approximately 2:30 a.m. burnt it under a bridge using diesel and petrol purchased for the purpose. Her scooter was discovered ten kilometres (6.2 miles) from where her body was found. Near the toll booth, officers discovered her clothes, handbag, boots, and a liquor bottle. The burns covered 70% of the body. A Ganesha locket discovered on the burnt body assisted her relatives in identifying the victim. After the post-mortem, the body was returned to the family.

INVESTIGATION

Four men were arrested by the police because of evidence from **CCTV** cameras and the victim's phone. The accused was taken into judicial custody at **Cherlapally Central Jail** for seven days. The Chief Minister of Telangana ordered a special court to quickly try them for their alleged crimes. A terrible rape and murder caused anger across the country. People held protests and demonstrations demanding stricter laws against rape and rapists. The Home Affairs Minister criticised the Telangana Police and insisted the government to amend the Indian Penal Code and Code of Criminal Procedure to instantly punish the criminals for their crimes through special courts. **On December 6, 2019**, all four accused men were killed while in police custody under a bridge on the Bengaluru-Hyderabad national highway. The police claimed that they were taken there to recreate the crime scene, but two of them supposedly grabbed guns and attacked the police. In the resulting exchange of gunfire, all four suspects were fatally shot. Some people accused the police of killing them without a fair trial, while hundreds of thousands of people celebrated the men's deaths.

After the four accused men were killed in the encounter, the first post-mortem was done on the same day at a government hospital in **Mahbubnagar**. Their bodies were then taken to Gandhi Hospital. Later, **on December 21**, the Telangana High Court ordered a second post-mortem. This second examination was carried out by forensic experts from AIIMS, Delhi, at a hospital in Hyderabad. After the second post-mortem, the bodies were given to their families after the identification process was completed.

In 2022, an Inquiry commission appointed by the Supreme Court of India reported that the encounter was likely staged, and the matter was transferred to the Telangana High Court for further action. The names of the four suspects who were killed in the encounter were **Mr. Chinta Kunta Chennakeshavulu, Mr. Jolu Shiva, Mr. Jollu Naveen, and Mr. Mohammed Arif.**

THE VICTIM

THE VICTIM Ms. DISHA (changed name to protect the identity) had pursued a degree in a veterinary college in Rajendranagar mandal. She was a resident of Shamshabad and was working as a veterinary assistant surgeon at the state-run hospital in Kollur village.

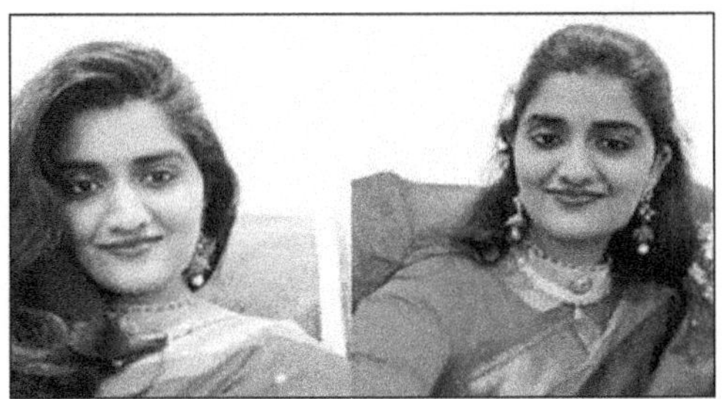

AFTERMATH

The family of the victim in Hyderabad, India, claims that the police should have responded more quickly and prevented her death. The police were not serious and proceeded with the case by improperly questioning the victim's family. They were sent to Thondupally toll plaza to conduct a search but were unsuccessful. Three police officers from the Shamshabad airport police station were suspended due to negligence and delay in filing a missing person's report. The local police convinced the victim's family to use a fictional name, Ms. Disha, to hide the victim's identity during media reporting and suggested using the hashtag **#JusticeForDisha** for social media posts to create awareness. Indian laws prohibit naming rape victims, and violations can result in legal penalties. In December, a man from Nizamabad district was arrested by the Hyderabad police for posting derogatory posts about the victim.

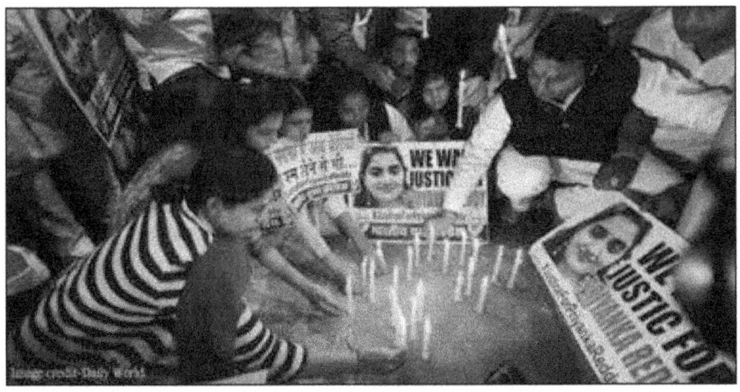

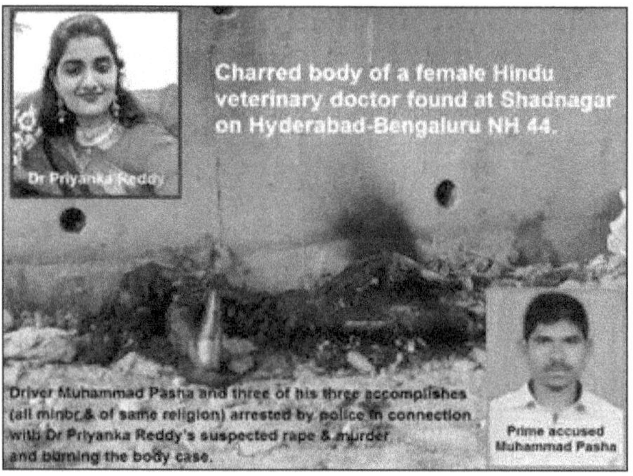

SECOND CORPSE

As of the first day of December 2019, the case is being investigated after the body of another woman was discovered nearby, half-burnt. According to the authorities, it was unclear whether she lit herself on fire or whether it was an accident. The veterinary's murder and the second corpse are unrelated, according to police.

PROTEST

India experienced widespread outrage following the rape and murder of four suspects, primarily in Hyderabad. The incident occurred near Rajiv Gandhi International Airport, and politicians like Mr. Rahul Gandhi expressed dismay. Protests called for stronger legislation to combat rape. The accused was placed under judicial custody for **14 days** due to a crowd of protestors surrounding the police station. Demonstrators threw stones at police cars as they moved the accused from Shadnagar to Hyderabad prison. The crowd demanded the police turn over the accused, leading to the police using force and batons to subdue them. The public had a negative opinion of the police, and demonstrators demanded their top objectives and urged them to behave proactively, sensitively, and responsively.

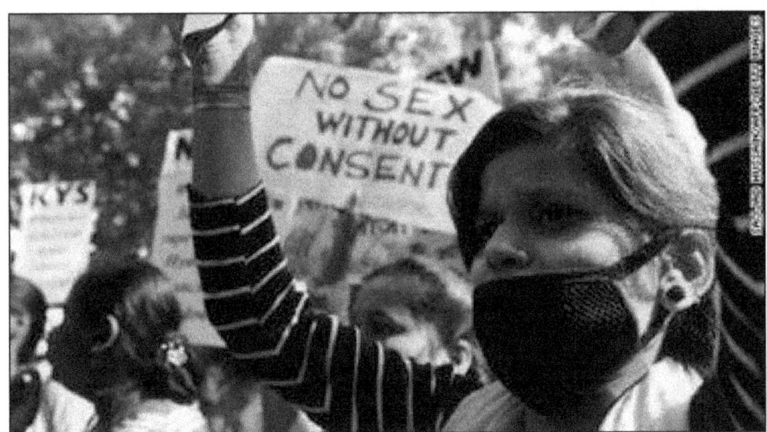

DISCUSSION IN PARLIAMENT

In December 2019, a serious incident was discussed in the Indian parliament. Members of both the Lok Sabha and Rajya Sabha were shocked by it and called for SWIFT ACTION. Government officials, like Mr. Rajnath Singh and Mr. G. Kishan Reddy, expressed their commitment to investigate and change laws to address such heinous crimes. Chairman Mr. Venkaiah Naidu allowed discussion about the incident but did not adjourn the session. During a heated debate, some members suggested harsh punishments like **lynching** and **castration** for convicted rapists to deter future offenders. They also demanded quick trials and the death penalty for the accused. Some members, like Mr. Mohd. Ali Khan emphasised the need for fast-track trials without bringing religion into the discussion. Even members who typically oppose the death penalty, like Mr. Binoy Viswam from the Communist Party of India, believed that these accused should be hanged due to the severity of the crime.

PROPOSED LEGAL CHANGES

During an **NDTV (NEW DELHI TELEVISION LTD)** interview, Union Minister of State for Home Mr. G. Kishan Reddy criticised the Telangana Police for their lack of urgency in responding to a crime and their casual attitude when dealing with victims. He emphasised the need for every police station to accept complaints without turning anyone away, with the option to file an FIR later. Reddy expressed a commitment to amend the Indian Penal Code (**IPC**) and Code of Criminal Procedure (**CrPC**) to ensure quicker punishment through fast-track courts. These changes were set to be discussed in a meeting of senior police officers **(DGPs)** between December 6 and 8. In addition to this, **the Bureau of Police Research and Development** (BPR&D) offered further suggestions for revisions to the IPC and CrPC rules. Furthermore, the Andhra Pradesh government passed a bill known as the **Disha Act (Andhra Pradesh Criminal Law (Amendment) Bill, 2019)**. This bill aimed to impose the death penalty on rapists within 21 days of the crime and sought to expedite the legal process. The goal was to publicise the use of the emergency response system **"112"** and encourage women to download the associated app for use in case of emergencies. This system would alert the police, law enforcement authorities, the victim's family, and even volunteers to ensure a swift response.

KILLING OF THE SUSPECT

All four accused were killed by the police in an encounter **on 6th December 2019**, under a bridge on the Bangalore-Hyderabad highway. This incident raised concerns of extrajudicial execution, meaning the police taking the law into their own hands.

According **to Deputy Commissioner Mr. Prakash Reddy of Shamshabad Police in Hyderabad**, the four suspects were taken to the location to re-enact the crime scene. However, two of them allegedly grabbed guns and attacked the police. In the resulting shootout, all four suspects were fatally shot. Reports in "The Indian Express" mentioned that the police claimed one of the accused signalled to the others to flee after the attack. The suspects tried to escape, and police fired in what they said was self-defence. The suspects were not handcuffed, and the police chief, Mr. V. C. Sajjanar, explained that the suspects were able to take and use the weapons because the guns were not locked. He stated that the suspects had attacked the police, and the officers responded which acted as self-defence.

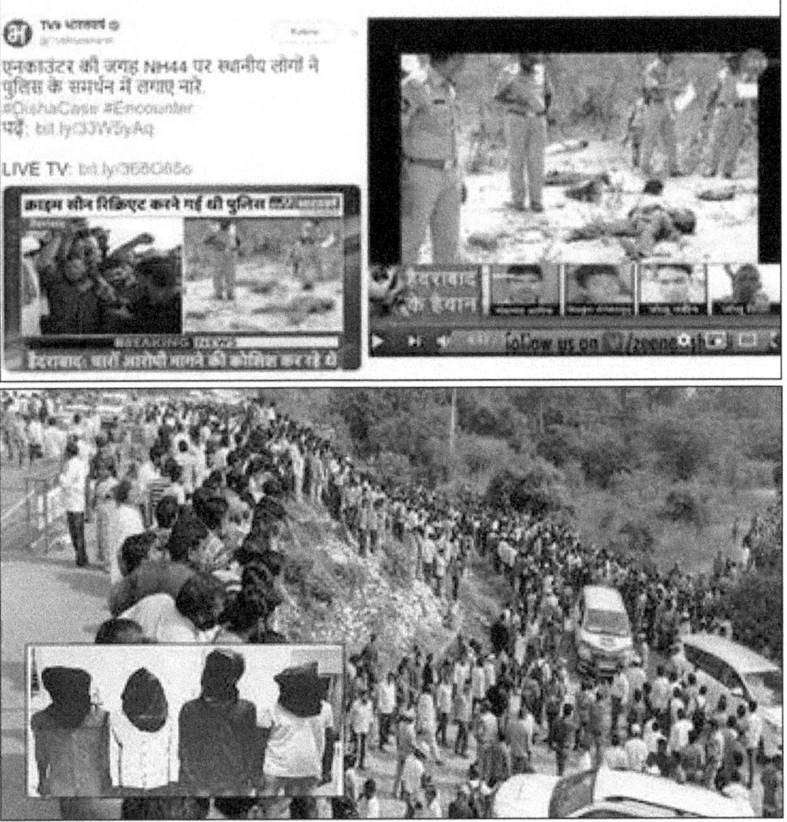

RESPONSE

In **December 2019**, four men accused of a heinous crime in India were killed by the police. Some people, including the victims' family, celebrated the police action, while others, like the families of the accused and human rights activists, were upset and criticised it.

The celebrations were due to frustration with the slow legal system in India, which often takes a long time to resolve cases. Some movies and social media posts also glorified police taking the law into their own hands. On the other hand, the families of the accused and many human rights organisations condemned the police encounter, saying it should have been handled in a court of law. They were concerned that the accused might have been innocent and now no one would ever know. Amnesty International called it an **"alleged extrajudicial execution"** and demanded an independent investigation. The National Human Rights Commission of India initiated an investigation, and in **May 2022**, the commission concluded that the encounter was staged, and the police deliberately intended to kill the accused. They recommended that the involved police officers be enquired for the murder. The Supreme Court of India transferred the matter to the Telangana High Court for further action.

LEGACY

In response to the incident, the Andhra Pradesh Legislative Assembly passed Andhra Pradesh Disha-Criminal Law **(Andhra Pradesh Amendment)** Bill, 2019 and Special Courts for **(Specified Offences against women and children)** Bill, 2020. The bills seek to expedite the investigation and trial of heinous cases related to sexual offences against women and children when substantial conclusive evidence is present. As of **July 2021**, the bills were reserved for the President's assent. In **September 2020**, filmmaker Mr. Ram Gopal Varma announced the film Disha Encounter, which is based on the incident. The Central Board of Film Certification initially refused to certify the film but later passed it with an adult-only rating. The film's release has been delayed by the **COVID-19 pandemic**, and the victim's parents approached the Telangana High Court petitioning that the film would bring disrepute to their family.

CONCLUSION

The Hyderabad rape involves the gang rape and murder of a veterinarian in Hyderabad, India, in November 2019. The incident sparked widespread outrage and protests across the country. The four accused individuals were arrested, and the case was fast-tracked through the Indian legal system. In December 2019, all four accused were killed in a police encounter while allegedly trying to escape during a crime scene reconstruction. This encounter was met with mixed reactions from the public.

SOURCES & REFERENCES

- Ganeshan, Balakrishna (29 November 2019). "When will our country be safe for Women?". The News Minute. Retrieved 30 November 2019.

- "3 policemen suspended for FIR delay in vet case". The Hindu. 30 November 2019. Retrieved 9 December 2019.

- Jump up to: Deshpande, Abhinay (3 December 2019). "Nizamabad youth held for vulgar posts about Hyderabad vet on Facebook". The Hindu. Retrieved 3 December 2019.

- Pavan, P. (1 December 2019). "Hyderabad rape and murder case: Cops change victim's name to 'Disha'". Pune Mirror. Mumbai Mirror. Retrieved 1 December 2019.

- "Hyderabad: Man arrested for objectionable Facebook posts on rape victim". Telangana Today. 3 December 2019. Retrieved 3 December 2019

Chapter 11

AARUSHI TALWAR AND HEMRAJ BANJADE: DOUBLE MURDER MYSTERY

Jaspreet Singh and Nikunj P. R.

ABSTRACT

In the tranquil neighbourhood of Noida, a chilling murder sent shockwaves throughout the nation, enthralling the public's imagination and baffling investigators. The Aarushi Talwar case, often referred to as the Noida double murder, where a 13-year-old girl was found brutally murdered in her own home in 2008, is a true crime episode that has ignited a decade-long saga filled with controversies. With gripping storytelling and meticulous research, this chapter seeks to unravel the layers of this complex, real-life thriller. This chapter is more than just a regurgitation of facts but an exploration of the limitations of Forensic Science and the role played by the media in high-profile cases. It looks at the various theories and speculations that have swirled around the Aarushi Talwar case, inviting readers to question: Who really killed Miss Aarushi?

KEYWORDS

Double Murder: Aarushi, Hemraj, Talwars

INTRODUCTION

In the suburban city of Noida, an unforgettable incident took place on 15 May 2008, as 13-year-old Miss Aarushi Talwar's life was brutally cut short, her skull cracked open, and throat brutally slit in the confines of her bedroom. To make the incident more confounding, 45-year-old worker Mr. Hemraj Benjade, who was considered the primary suspect, was found dead the next day on the terrace of the Talwar family's residence. The signs of sexual intercourse between the two, an adolescent and a middle-aged man, only served to highlight the case, causing it to become a nationwide sensation. The core of this investigation was Aarushi's parents, Dr. Rajesh and Dr. Nupur Talwar, who were caught up in a turbulent web of court cases, as the police suspected them of the double murder. The dramatic media attention, in addition to dealing with the pain of losing their beloved daughter, pitied them.

A bewildering mix of allegations, including a botched investigation and even suggestions of extramarital affairs, caused the case to be taken over by the Central Bureau of Intelligence (CBI), who then suspected the Talwars' assistant Mr. Krishna Thadarai and two domestic servants—Mr. Rajkumar and Mr. Vijay Mandal. Unconventional, illegal scientific tests were conducted on them, and although no concrete evidence regarding who had committed the double homicide was acquired, it was concluded that Dr. Rajesh Talwar was not involved and was set free 50 days after his arrest. However, the CBI's methods and the validity of these confessions soon came under scrutiny.

In 2009, the case was handed over to a new team leading to a recommendation to close the investigation. This new team identified Dr. Rajesh Talwar as the only suspect based on circumstantial evidence but declined to prosecute him because of the significant gaps in the evidence. The Talwars objected to the closure report, claiming that Dr. Rajesh Talwar's suspicions by the CBI were unfounded, sparking a legal battle that would redefine their fate. Dramatic turns occurred in the ensuing legal processes, with a special CBI court dismissing the agency's claim of inadequate evidence and launching charges against the Talwars. In a harrowing verdict delivered in November 2013, Miss Arushi's parents were found guilty and sentenced to life imprisonment, amid a chorus of criticism that the judgement was based on flimsy grounds. In 2017, the Allahabad High Court acquitted the Talwar family, bringing an end to their harrowing ordeal. Yet despite all this, the case remains unsolved.

THE FAMILY

- Dr. Rajesh Talwar and Dr. Nupur Talwar were Miss Aarushi Talwar's parents, dentists who lived in Noida, Uttar Pradesh, and were in their forties. They were both convicted of the murder of their only daughter, Miss Aarushi, and their live-in house helper, Mr. Hemraj Banjade.

- Dr. Dinesh Talwar, Rajesh Talwar's elder brother, and Dr. Vandana Talwar, the wife of Mr. Dinesh Talwar.

- Group Captain (Retd) Mr. Bhalachandra Chitnis and his wife, Mrs. Lata, were Nupur's parents living in the same suburb as Rajesh and Nupur.

THE FRIENDS

- Mr. Ajay Chaddha was a businessman and a close family friend of the Talwar family.

- Dr Praful and Dr Anita Durrani were close family friends, living in Noida. They used to spend most of their holidays with the Talwar family. Mr. Rajkumar, one of the suspects in this case, was working under them.

- Miss Vidushi Durrani and Miss Fiza Jha were Miss Aarushi's friends and schoolmates. Vidushi is Mr. Praful's and Mrs. Anita's daughter.

THE VICTIMS

- Miss Aarushi Talwar, a bright and cheerful 13-year-old studying at Delhi Public School in Noida, Uttar Pradesh. Her dead body was found at her own residence, her throat slit open, and her head struck by an object.

- Mr. Hemraj Banjade, a 45-year-old Nepalese man working as a live-in house helper for the Talwar family. His dead body was found on the terrace of the Talwars' home on the very next day after Miss Aarushi's death.

TALWAR'S FAMILY BACKGROUND

After Miss Aarushi was born, Dr. Rajesh and Dr. Nupur moved to Jalvayu Vihar, located in Noida, because Dr. Nupur's parents lived in the same complex, and the Talwars needed some support from their grandparents for Miss Aarushi's upbringing. Dr. Rajesh and Dr. Nupur were dentists beginning to make a name for themselves in society. As Miss Aarushi grew up, she was a bright student and was studying at Delhi Public School. The place where the Talwars moved was a suburban housing society built in the '90s and was allotted to Air Force or Navy officers. As time passed, the area became home to four thousand flats and ten thousand residents. It was a middle-class settlement housing colony, where servants used to come to most of the flats for work, and in the rarest of cases, someone would keep a live-in house helper. The Talwars had a regular maid named Ms. Kalpana and a live-in house helper, Mr. Hemraj.

BODIES DISCOVERED

On the morning of 16th May 2008, Ms. Kalpana was on leave and found Ms. Bharti as a replacement. Ms. Bharti rang the doorbell, but no one responded. She pressed the doorbell again and went to take the mop and bucket that were usually kept on the stairs of the terrace near the house entrance. It was Mr. Hemraj's work to open the door, but he did not respond. Dr. Nupur woke up to the doorbell and came to the inner door of the flat.

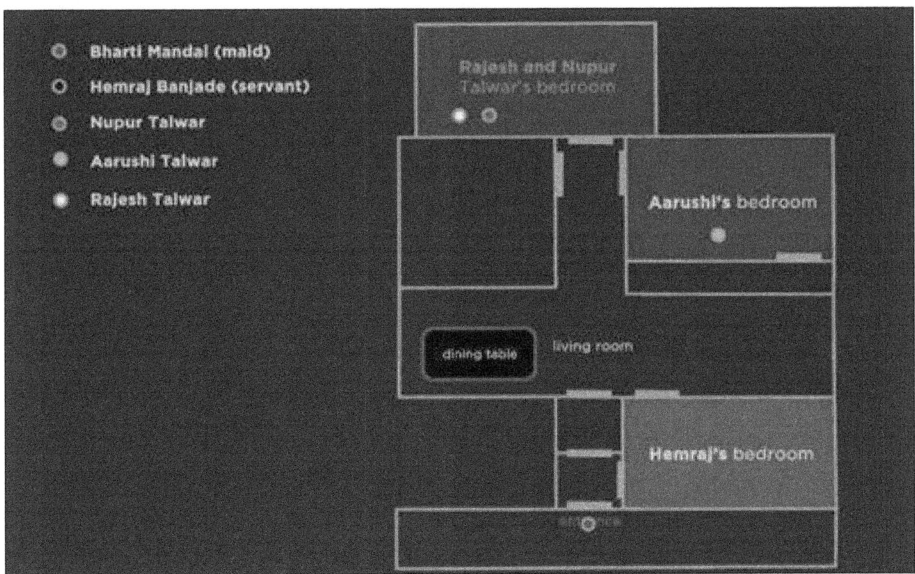

To enter the Talwars' flat, there were three doors. The outermost door was an iron grill door which opened to a short passage. After the passage, there were two doors built into the same frame. On the outer side, there was a mesh door, and behind it was a wooden door with a mortise lock that would open into the drawing room. Having a mortise lock on the wooden door states that no one can enter the flat without the key because a mortise lock allows the opening of the door from the inside, but to enter from the outside, a key is necessary. The mesh door, on the other hand, has a normal latch; entry can be from the inside or outside too.

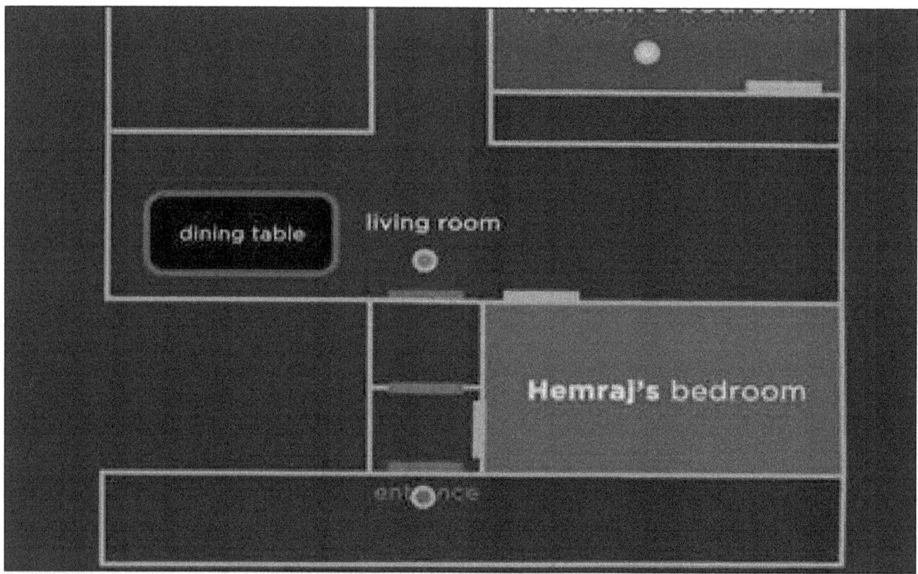

As Dr. Nupur unlocked the wooden door, she found the mesh door locked from the outside. She told Ms. Bharti that Mr. Hemraj might have gone to get milk and suggested she come to the balcony and catch the key for the mesh door she would be throwing from the balcony so that she could come into the house. By the time Dr. Rajesh Talwar woke up, he walked to the drawing room and found Ballantine's Scotch whisky on the dining table. The entire family slept around 11:30, and the previous night no one had drunk, and this frightened him. Dr. Nupur, too, did not know about the bottle being on the dining table.

They saw Miss Aarushi's bedroom door was partially open as they went towards the bedroom. Miss Aarushi's dead body was lying on her own bed covered with a white blanket, her pillow and mattress covered with blood which was dripping to the floor. Heartbreaking, isn't it? Seeing your own kid's dead body who was about to turn fourteen in a few days. The night before Miss Aarushi's death, Dr. Rajesh and Dr. Nupur gave Miss Aarushi an early birthday present, a Sony 10-megapixel digital camera. After giving the present to Miss Aarushi, Dr. Rajesh and Dr. Nupur went to their room, Dr. Rajesh had some work to continue on his laptop and so Dr. Nupur went to Miss Aarushi's room to switch on the router. She saw Miss Aarushi reading a book, "The Three Mistakes of My Life" by Chetan Bhagat. The next morning, she saw Miss Aarushi's dead body in Miss Aarushi's bedroom. Dr. Nupur lifted the blanket and saw their only daughter's throat had been slit open with a sharp object and her skull just above the forehead struck by a blunt object. By the time Ms. Bharti came upstairs, she found a latch on the mesh door. Undoing the latch, she entered the flat and found Dr. Nupur and Dr. Rajesh crying, with a shocked and bewildered reaction. She went to Miss Aarushi's bedroom along with Dr. Nupur and saw her dead body. Later, Ms. Bharti informed the neighbours and the security guard, who called the police.

Later, Dr. Rajesh and Dr. Nupur informed this to three couples close to them: Dr. Nupur's parents, Dr. Rajesh's brother and his wife, and the Durranis, who were their close friends, and their daughter, Miss Vidushi, was Miss Aarushi's closest friend. When they all arrived, all were in a state of shock and could say nothing. As the news of Miss Aarushi's death was spreading, within an hour, Talwar's flat was filled with policemen, media, neighbours, etc. It was a crime scene where there were more than twenty people; no efforts were made by the police to secure the crime scene, which led to the disturbance of many pieces of evidence. Despite all that, police started the initial examination of the scene as a kick-start for the investigation. There were no signs of forced entry, no sign of theft, and nothing like a murder weapon was found. Upon examination of Miss Aarushi's room, they saw some dress and a blanket over Miss Aarushi's body, making it look like she was still sleeping. The bedroom was not the only place where the police found blood. The scotch bottle kept on the dining table had some fingerprints with blood stains, and those fingerprints were not identified. The presence of the scotch bottle on the dining table with the fingerprints states that the perpetrator knew the place where the bottle was kept and knew the house very well. The presence of blood-stained fingerprints on the bottle reveals that the perpetrator had enough time to stay in the house without the fear of being caught after murdering Miss Aarushi. Later, police found blood stains on the stairs that led to the terrace locked door. The police were not the first ones to locate those stains; some friends of Dr. Rajesh saw these and brought them to the authorities' attention, theorising that the perpetrator might have used it as a path to run. The key to unlocking the terrace door could not be located, so they diverted their attention from the terrace.

Everybody was present at the scene, but Mr. Hemraj, the live-in house helper, was missing. Dr. Nupur called Mr. Hemraj; the call was connected but there was silence for a few seconds, after which the person on the other side hung up. Immediately, Dr. Nupur suspected that Mr. Hemraj might have murdered Miss Aarushi and fled. Dr. Rajesh Talwar then dictated an FIR against Mr. Hemraj, suspecting him of the murder of Miss Aarushi. The search for Mr. Hemraj began, and there were some pre-cremation rituals and an autopsy that needed to be taken care of.

Miss Aarushi's body was sent for autopsy. The report states that nothing abnormal was detected with the injuries. Miss Aarushi's vaginal swabs were also tested for rape or any sexual assaults that happened to her. The report did not suggest any signs of rape or sexual assault with Miss Aarushi. The same day, the cremation of Ms. Aarushi was done. The house was in a mess, and a few ladies cleaned the house. Protocols were not followed as the police kept neglecting the evidence; they did not even care to find a locksmith who could unlock the terrace door.

The next morning, Dr. Rajesh and Dr. Nupur were leaving for Haridwar to immerse Miss Aarushi's ashes. On the way, Mr. Dinesh Talwar, the elder brother of Dr. Rajesh Talwar, informed Dr. Rajesh that a body was found on the terrace. Without any delay, Dr. Rajesh and Dr. Nupur returned to Jalvayu Vihar. Dr. Rajesh went upstairs to identify the body while Dr. Nupur waited outside the building with Miss Aarushi's remains. That same morning, Mr. KK Gautam, a retired police officer who helped speed up Miss Aarushi's autopsy, arrived at the Talwar's house to offer his condolences. He then decided to investigate the case on his own. Mr. Gautam discovered blood stains leading to the terrace since there was no key, as the officer demanded yesterday. Therefore, with the help of local police, he broke the lock on the terrace door and entered the terrace. In the hot sun, a body was found in a decaying condition on the terrace, and it still had a slipper on it. The dead body was half covered with a cooler panel and a bedsheet had been hung on the other side to prevent anyone from noticing the body. The blood stains belonging to the person were unidentified.

On 17th May 2008, Mr. Hemraj's body was discovered by Mr. KK Gautam and identified by Dr. Rajesh Talwar. The prime suspect of the case was found dead, and the case has again turned back to the same point where it all started. The difference was the number of dead bodies; previously, it was only Miss Aarushi's, but now there's Mr. Hemraj too. Later, a post-mortem analysis states that Mr. Hemraj was also hit by a heavy blunt object on his head, and his throat was slit open with a sharp object. It was the same way Miss Aarushi was murdered, and the estimated time of death (TOD) was also the same as Miss Aarushi's. As many people were gathered on the terrace, they identified a handprint covered with blood by the door side. It was assumed to be Mr. Hemraj's handprint, but identification of the handprint was not successful because it was partially smudged, and it was too late for the fingerprints to be lifted off. Due to this, the police's ability to solve this case was heavily criticised. After all this, the police failed to follow the protocol, secure the crime scene, conduct a proper search, secure the evidence, and many more things that could have solved the case.

On 21st May 2008, Delhi police were involved in the investigation to lead it in the right direction. As Miss Aarushi's family was living in a modern suburban area, they had given phones to both Miss Aarushi to call and chat with her friends and family, and Mr. Hemraj was given the phone for work purposes, but both the phones were missing after that night. The police obtained the call records of both phones. Mr. Hemraj's calls were for work purposes, mostly from Talwar's clinic, but the last call was at 8:27 pm the night before the incident; he received a call from the PCO that lasted about six minutes. Miss Aarushi's phone was only for texting and calling her friends, so there was not anything unusual among them. There was a boy named 'Anmol' who was Miss Aarushi's boyfriend in the month prior to her murder. Police theorised that he might know something about Miss Aarushi's personal life and interests.

On 22nd May 2008, Mr. Anmol was brought in for interrogation. There, he stated that he was on a call with Miss Aarushi prior to her murder, and Miss Aarushi had told him about the affair that Dr. Rajesh Talwar was having with his colleague, Anita Durrani. The police then echoed this information in front of the media with their theory of the double murder of Miss Aarushi and Mr. Hemraj. The police stated the extramarital affairs that Miss Aarushi knew about and that were going on between Dr. Rajesh Talwar and Dr. Anita Durrani. Miss Aarushi would discuss this with Mr. Hemraj, and this discussion brought them together. They also stated that, on that night, Dr. Rajesh found Mr. Hemraj and Miss Aarushi in Miss Aarushi's room, where he saw both in an objectionable state but not in a compromising position. Dr. Rajesh took Mr. Hemraj to the terrace for a talk, and there he murdered him. After that, he returned to have a drink and then killed Miss Aarushi. This piece of information blew up the media, and it turned against the parents. This led to the arrest of Miss Aarushi's father, Dr. Rajesh Talwar, on 23rd May 2008.

The media had several questions for the parents; amongst them, the media asked if the parents had heard anything from Miss Aarushi's room that night, claiming that there was only a plywood partition between the two rooms. To this, Dr. Rajesh Talwar said that it was not a plywood partition; it was a wall made of brick with a plywood lamination over it, and the two Air Conditioners were switched on that night. He also mentioned that the two doors were closed which were made of wood. On top of that, Miss Aarushi had a throat infection so she could not scream loudly. This scene was also reconstructed and tested in the same room under the same condition to confirm the accused. The result of the reconstruction stated that no sound was made travelling from Miss Aarushi's room to Dr. Rajesh and Dr. Nupur's room.

Another question raised by the media was the objectionable position in which Dr. Rajesh found Miss Aarushi and Mr. Hemraj together. It was denied by the lack of blood present on their pyjamas. The next morning, Dr. Nupur Talwar stated that no parent would kill their own child. Questions on the affair between Dr. Rajesh and Dr. Anita were also denied by Dr. Nupur Talwar, who claimed that they were an "extended family".

In continuation, more questions were also raised about misleading the police about Miss Aarushi's parents to find Mr. Hemraj instead of searching the flat. The media claimed that they were trying to put an end to the further investigation and confused it. The Talwars strongly denied it and told the media that they were randomly assuming as they found their only daughter murdered and since Mr. Hemraj was also missing, they suspected Mr. Hemraj to be the possible murderer. Transferring the case to Delhi police made the situation even worse. This led to destroying the reputation of the family and judging Miss Aarushi's personal life as a 'characterless girl'. Miss Aarushi's character assassination and the destruction of the family's reputation reached the ears of the Chief Minister of Uttar Pradesh, Ms. Mayawati, and she transferred the case to the Central Bureau of Investigation (CBI). Then, on 31st May 2008, the CBI took over and investigated the case of Aarushi Talwar and Hemraj Banjade's Murder.

THE INVESTIGATION

Once the case was taken over by the CBI from the local police, the CBI's forensic team re-examined the crime scene and collected the leftover evidence. While this was going on, Mr. Arun Kumar, head of the investigating CBI team, made an inventory of the investigative blunders that had occurred so far. As he was going through the statements collected by the police, he realised that it was Mr. Krishna Thadarai who insinuated the idea that Dr. Rajesh was an adulterer and debauch, who had an affair with his colleague Dr. Anita Durrani. However, when Miss Aarushi found out, she sought comfort in Mr. Hemraj's arms.

On 1st July 2008, Mr. K.K. Gautham said he did a formal inspection of Mr. Hemraj's room, where he found depressions in the mattress from which he concluded three people may have sat on it. He also observed three glasses, two still containing some amounts of liquor, and a whisky bottle which was a quarter full. He also inspected the toilets and deduced that more than one person had used them. He found that fingerprints of the Talwars were not present on the whisky bottle. This suggested the presence of outsiders that night.

Mr. Arun felt that Mr. Krishna Thadarai had to be interrogated once more. On June 7th, Mr. Krishna was detained on suspicion. When the CBI checked his house, they found a pillowcase with a drop of Mr. Hemraj's blood, along with a blood-stained kukri and trousers. Mr. Krishna was subjected to a polygraph test conducted by the then head of CFSL, Dr. Bibha Rani Ray. Behavioural scientists present at the time described him as deceptive and quick to shift the blame onto others. A few days after this test, he was subjected to a narcoanalysis test, which, although the forceful use of it is considered a violation of fundamental human rights, if significant evidence is obtained via voluntary testing, can be admissible in court. He spilled the beans on the details of the crime and the weapon used. He talked about two other servants who were present at the house that day along with Mr. Hemraj - Mr. Raj Kumar and Mr. Vijay Mandal. He said he saw Mr. Raj Kumar committing the murder and that Mr. Rajesh had nothing to do with it, but due to the inconsistencies in his story and attempts at deception, the CBI did not take this as integral evidence. The medical professionals who performed Miss Aarushi's autopsy, Dr. Sunil Dohre and Dr. Naresh Raj, gave new statements when questioned by the CBI. According to them, Miss Aarushi's hymen was ruptured, and it looked like her privates had been cleansed. According to Dr. Naresh Raj, Mr. Hemraj's enlarged penis indicated the possibility of sexual intercourse. In October 2009, a crime scene analysis was done by the CBI based on the photographs of the scene, which supported the conjecture that the crime scene had been dressed up after the murders.

Since there was no indication of forced entry into the residence and no known motive, the CBI ruled out the involvement of any other intruders other than Mr. Krishna, Mr. Rajkumar, and Mr. Mandal. Furthermore, the CBI said that an outsider would not have tried to conceal Mr. Hemraj's body by dragging it and covering it with a cooler panel or dressing up the crime scene.

The CBI said that the circumstantial evidence suggested that the parents were involved in the crime. They felt that the Talwars were the only ones with the reason and the ability to dress up the crime scene. According to the CBI, the wounds on Miss Aarushi's neck were "surgical" and could only have been performed by qualified professionals, to which they fit the part. Also, the blunt injury on her head seemed to have been caused by a golf club. After a period of investigation, the CBI submitted a closure report in the case, which basically recommended closing the investigation without pressing charges against the Talwars. However, the court rejected the closure report and initiated court proceedings against the Talwars. The case proceeded to trial, which led to the Talwars' conviction and subsequent appeal.

THE FINAL VERDICT OF THE CASE

On 25 November 2013, a special CBI court in Ghaziabad, India, delivered its verdict in the case and held Dr. Rajesh and Dr. Nupur Talwar guilty of the two murders. The Special Judge Shyam Lal convicted the couple for the following: murder, destruction of evidence, misleading the probe, and filing a wrong FIR. On 26 November 2013, they were sentenced to life imprisonment for the twin murders of their daughter Miss Arushi and the domestic help Mr. Hemraj.

The Talwar family called the verdict a 'miscarriage of justice' and alleged that points proving the innocence of Dr. Rajesh and Dr. Nupur were not produced by the CBI. Journalist Mr. Avirook Sen alleged that the Judge wrote the case verdict even before the defence side had finished their arguments. Nonetheless, the Talwars filed an appeal against the trial court's ruling with the Allahabad High Court. In October 2017, The Allahabad High Court reversed the Talwars' conviction and acquitted them. The court determined that the evidence was insufficient to prove their guilt beyond a reasonable doubt. The High Court's verdict highlighted the importance of a fair and thorough investigation and the need for substantial evidence to convict.

The Allahabad High Court's acquittal of the Talwars marked the final verdict in the Aarushi Talwar double murder case. It brought an end to a legal battle that spanned several years and had been the subject of intense public interest and media scrutiny.

DOUBLE MURDER MYSTERY

Initially, the police considered that the Talwars had murdered their daughter in a fit of rage upon discovering Miss Aarushi in a compromising position with Mr. Hemraj. This was essentially done with the intention of protecting the family's honour. Another theory was that Dr. Rajesh was having an affair with his friend and co-worker, Dr. Anita Durrani, and when Miss Aarushi found out, she sought comfort in Mr. Hemraj's arms, which when discovered by Dr. Rajesh caused him to go on a rampage and kill them both. There were also speculations about a burglary that escalated into murder. Some believed that intruders had broken into their house to steal valuables but encountered Miss Aarushi and Mr. Hemraj, which led to their tragic ending. Although there are multiple theories such as the ones mentioned above and others, such as it was committed by the workers - Mr. Krishna Thadarai, Mr. Rajkumar, and Mr. Vijay Mandal under the influence of alcohol, it did not hold as there was no motive for them to do so. The outsiders did not show traits a criminal did, like hiding or not showing up for interrogation.

It also did not make sense for Mr. Krishna to have been the one who did it as there was no incriminating evidence found against him. It was also not possible for him to have hidden the body on the terrace, while the area was secured and surrounded by the police. This case has continued to remain a mystery for the past decade with no leads on who committed the double homicide.

CONTROVERSIES AND PUBLIC OPINION

A lot of controversies surrounded the initial investigation conducted by the police. There was no effort from their side to barricade the crime scene, causing visitors to conduct their own investigations.

They also did not find a locksmith to open the locked terrace for a whole day. Critics alleged that the vital evidence was mishandled, lost or tampered with, leading to a flawed investigation.

Other theories were surrounding the Talwars. Although it is improbable for a parent to kill their child, it is not impossible. Questions were raised on how the couple could have slept through a violent, bloody, gruesome double murder involving their child while living under the same roof. The use of narcoanalysis tests on the suspects - The Talwars and Mr. Krishna Thadarai - drew significant controversy. Many questioned the ethics, admissibility, and reliability of evidence obtained through this controversial technique. The CBI's investigation was filled with shifting theories and suspect narratives. They later submitted a closure report recommending closing the investigation due to lack of evidence, but the CBI later initiated proceedings against the Talwars. This brought up questions regarding the authenticity of the investigation.

In 2009, Miss Aarushi Talwar's vaginal swab sample was tampered with, leading to a conspiracy theory. The CBI sent the sample to a Delhi lab, where it was found to be a mix of two samples, one of which was Miss Aarushi's. The Centre for DNA Fingerprinting and Diagnostics (CDFD) in Hyderabad found the sample contained DNA of a person other than Miss Aarushi. The CBI concluded that the original sample was Miss Aarushi's, but it had become contaminated. The Talwars were questioned about the tampering allegations during their lie-detector and brain-mapping tests but were cleared. The incident was dismissed as a genuine mistake. The involvement of the media in this case was highly controversial. Despite raising awareness of the case, media coverage has drawn criticism for making the story a sensation, biased reporting, and played a pivotal role in shaping public opinion affecting the investigation's direction.

The intense media coverage led to a de facto trial by the media, where the case was argued, discussed, and judged in the public domain. The media's narrative often favoured one theory over another, impacting how the public perceived the case. The continuous speculations influenced the public's views, hindering the suspects from receiving a fair trial. The Talwars, in particular, were under intense scrutiny in the eyes of the public.

AFTERMATH

- The Indian police created new standards for investigating child-related offences. These standards mandate that all cases of child sexual abuse be investigated by specialised units and that all minors interrogated by police be accompanied by a parent or guardian.

- A number of new programmes have been launched by the Indian government to safeguard children against abuse. These programmes include abuse reporting hotlines and shelters for abused children.

- The Indian media has established new reporting criteria for crimes affecting minors. These rules include the restriction on identifying child abuse victims and the need for all child abuse reports to be attentive to the interests of children.

- In 2017, the Talwars were acquitted of the killings, but the case remains unsolved.

- The Talwars have launched a defamation complaint against the media for their portrayal of them throughout the trial.

- The case has also inspired a number of novels and films.

- Miss Aarushi has a number of monuments devoted to her memory. Her family's home in Noida has one monument. It's a tiny tree with the inscription "In loving memory of Aarushi Talwar." Another monument can be seen in Noida's Radha Krishna Temple. It is an Aarushi statue with the inscription "Aarushi: A light that will never be extinguished."

- In the United States, there is also a memorial to Miss Aarushi. It is situated on the campus of the University of Maryland, Baltimore County, where Miss Aarushi's parents studied dentistry. The monument is a bench with the inscription, "In loving memory of Aarushi Talwar, a beautiful and innocent child who was taken from us far too soon."

- The tributes to Miss Aarushi Talwar are a means to commemorate and honour her memory. They serve as a reminder of her tragic demise and the need to protect children from harm.

CONCLUSION

The Aarushi Talwar murder case continues to remain one of India's most perplexing and controversial unsolved crimes. Despite years of investigation and a sensational trial, the identities of Miss Aarushi and Mr. Hemraj's killer, and the motive behind their murders remain shrouded in mystery.

The initial investigation by the Noida police, marred by mishandling of evidence and premature conclusions, cast suspicion on Miss Aarushi's parents, Dr. Rajesh and Dr. Nupur Talwar. However, the Central Bureau of Investigation (CBI) took over the case and ultimately acquitted the Talwars, citing a lack of concrete evidence. The CBI's theory stated that domestic help Mr. Krishna Thadarai and two other servants were involved in the murders, which also crumbled due to a lack of supporting evidence. The investigation was further hampered by the destruction of crucial evidence during the initial police probe. As the years passed, the case grew cold, with no new leads or suspects emerging. The Talwars, despite being acquitted, bore the stigma of suspicion and continued to grapple with the loss of their daughter. Mr. Hemraj's family was also left without justice, their son's murder seemingly forgotten.

The murder of Miss Aarushi Talwar serves as a vivid reminder of India's criminal justice system's shortcomings, the devastating impact of violence on families, and the lingering pain of unsolved crimes. The case also presents important issues regarding the nature of evidence, the role of the media, and the presumption of the innocent. While the case may never be definitively resolved, the Aarushi Talwar murder case continues to haunt India's collective memory, a testament to the enduring power of unsolved crimes and the quest for justice.

SOURCES & REFERENCES

- Mishra, S. (2021). A Study of Direct Evidence and Circumstantial Evidence with Special Reference to Aarushi Talwar Case. *Issue 3 Int'l JL Mgmt. & Human.*, *4*, 950.

- https://en.wikipedia.org/wiki/2008_Noida_double_murder_case

Chapter 12

SURYANELLI RAPE CASE

Macthalin Reshma I, Harshini L and Glenda B George

ABSTRACT

A well-known occurrence that took place in the Indian state of Kerala in 1996 is the Suryanelli rape case. It concerned the 16-year-old girl who became known as the "Suryanelli girl" being kidnapped and sexually assaulted. She said forty-two guys kidnapped and sexually assaulted her over the course of 40 days. Because of its horrific nature and the participation of powerful people, the case attracted a lot of attention. The matter went through a protracted court process with several trials and rulings. The Kerala High Court cleared every accused person in 2005 after a special court had found 35 of them guilty at first. The Supreme Court stepped in as a result of the public uproar and demonstrations caused by this ruling. The Kerala High Court was instructed by the Supreme Court to reexamine the case before rendering a decision. In 2013, the Kerala High Court overturned its previous ruling, which led to Adv. Dharmarajan, the principal accused, being found guilty and other people being found not guilty.

The Suryanelli case continues to be a representation of the difficulties and complications involved in obtaining justice for victims of sexual assault, and it has influenced conversations regarding India's legal system and about the way these cases are being investigated.

KEYWORDS

Adv. Dharmarajan, Mr. P. J. Kurian, Kerala High Court, Janadhipatya Mahila Association, rape, kidnapping, Supreme Court.

INTRODUCTION

The 1996 abduction and subsequent rape of a 16-year-old schoolgirl from Suryanelli, Kerala, India, is known as the Suryanelli rape case (also known as the Suryanelli sex scandal). On January 16, 1996, the girl was allegedly abducted after being seduced with the promise of marriage. Over the course of 40 days, 37 out of the forty-two accused people are said to have raped her. The rest had helped to facilitate the crime. The matter became politicised because of an impending general election after Prof. P.J. Kurien, a former Union Minister and later the deputy chairman of the Rajya Sabha, was named. Prof. Kurien was a member of the UDF, which was run by the Congress party. The case has attracted the attention of numerous women's rights advocates, including Mrs. K. Ajitha and Mrs. Suja Susan George, as well as women's organisations, including NFIW and Anweshi.

A Special Court in Kottayam found 35 out of thirty-nine defendants who were put on trial guilty of a variety of offences on 2nd September 2000. The primary accused, Adv. Dharmarajan, was convicted of several counts on July 12, 2002, and given a life sentence. He did, however, vanish after being released from custody on bond on 25th October 2002. The Kerala High Court cleared all thirty-five of the convicted on 20th January 2005, with the exception of chief accused Adv. Dharmarajan, because there was insufficient evidence to support the victim's account. She was declared untrustworthy by the court. The High Court's acquittals were overturned, and a new hearing was mandated by the Supreme Court of India in January 2013. In a TV appearance at the beginning of February 2013, Adv. Dharmarajan said that Prof. P. J. Kurien was implicated and the police hushed it up. This caused a political rift, with MPs calling for Prof. Kurien's resignation. On April 4, 2007, the Kerala High Court cleared Prof. Kurien of all allegations. The Supreme Court also confirmed it. It caused a minor dispute in the Indian parliament as well. Adv. Dharmarajan was arrested not long after that. He recanted his earlier remarks in May. The Kerala High Court exonerated Prof. Kurien of all charges.

On April 4, 2014, the Kerala High Court cleared seven of the thirty-five remaining defendants and maintained Adv. Dharmarajan's life sentence. As of October 2015, the case was on appeal at the Supreme Court.

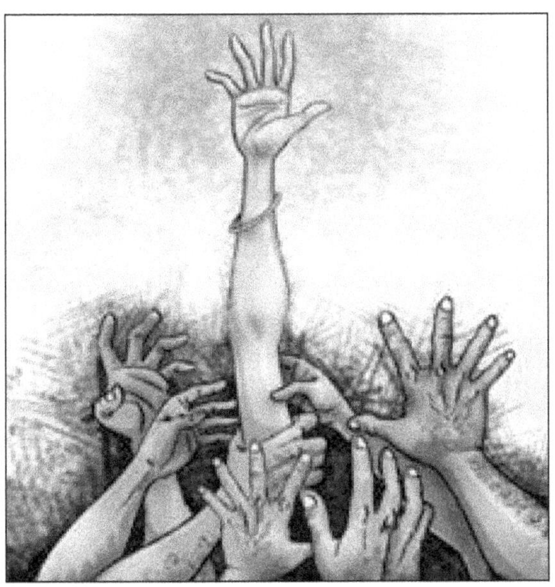

CASE INCIDENT

A 16-year-old girl from Suryanelli village in the Idukki district vanished from her hostel on January 16, 1996 (the initial report had her age listed as 15). The father, who works for the Department of Telecommunications, had been posted in Suryanelli, so the family came here. The girl was a student at Little Flower Convent School in Munnar and lived in the hostel there. Her father reported her missing, but she was never located despite a police search. Forty days later, on February 26, 1996, the girl was back at her father's place of employment. The following day, the police were notified of her kidnapping and rape.

INVESTIGATIONS

On February 28, 1996, the girl was examined by gynaecologist Dr. V. K. Bhaskaran (later prosecution witness #73) at Government Taluk Hospital, Adimali. He reported that the vulva was oedematous and that the vaginal exam hurt. The physician claimed that the victim had been the victim of "violent sexual acts" during the 2002 trial. Infection was present. According to the doctor, having sex while infected would have been uncomfortable. He said there was no laceration on the vaginal wall. Lacerations can occur during violent interactions. According to the physician, there was no indication or proof of resistance. "If, as stated by the victim, she was raped after being threatened and intimidated, then there would not be any sign of resistance on her body," the doctor said, not ruling out the possibility of rape. In addition to the victim's obvious distress, the infection, inflammation, ulcers, and new tears indicated violence. He also mentioned that, considering the timeframe, any abrasions or contusions sustained in the first few days would have healed by the end of the experience.

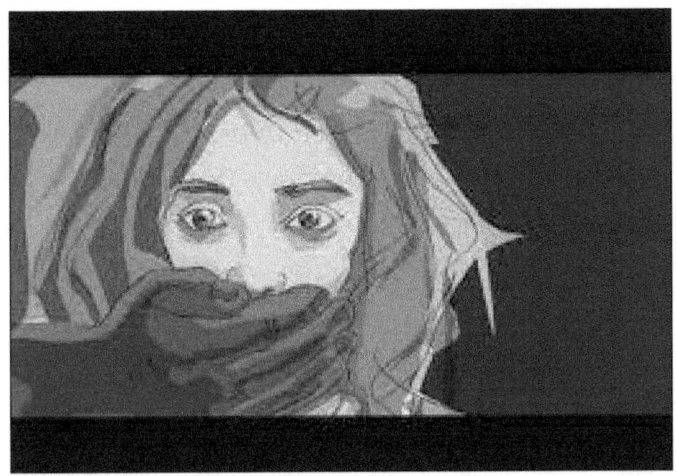

Forty of the initial forty-two suspects were located by 1999, according to the police. Lawmakers and other well-known individuals were on the list.

THE PROSECUTION'S ACCOUNT OF EVENTS

The prosecution found that she had been coaxed by a bus conductor, Mr. Raju (accused #1), to elope with him. On January 16, 1996, Mr. Raju asked the girl to leave her hostel in Munnar and meet him at Adimali. At 4:30 p.m., he persuaded her to travel with him to Kothamangalam. The man left the girl on the bus and got off in the middle. At 7:30 p.m., the girl arrived at her destination. She made the decision to continue to Kottayam, the home of her mother's sister. She travelled to Muvattupuzha by bus. She rode an autorickshaw to the KSRTC bus stop after arriving in Muvattupuzha. She then boarded a swift passenger bus headed for Trivandrum. She saw a woman on this bus who was later identified as Mrs. Usha (accused #2).

When she finally arrived in Kottayam, she was afraid to drive through the dark streets. She made the decision to visit her uncle in Mundakkayam. However, at night, there was no bus to Mundakkayam.

Mrs. Usha came up to her and said she could assist. She took the girl to Adv. Sreekumar, a lawyer and key culprit who was later identified as Adv. Dharmarajan. He vowed that he would take her to Mundakayam later. He informed her that she was welcome to stay at the resort where his mother was staying. The girl consented to go with him, but inside the lodge, he sexually assaulted her. Her father had reported her missing that same evening. After searching, an assistant sub-inspector was unable to find her.

The next morning, she was taken to Ernakulam on a bus. Thereafter, she was taken to various places, which included Kumili, Kambam, Palakkad, Vanimel, Aluva, Theni, Kanyakumari, Trivandrum, and Kuravilangad. On the morning of 26 February 1996, she was freed. During the intervening period, she was raped or gang-raped by thirty-eight out of the forty-two accused. The remaining four, including Mrs. Usha and Mr. Raju, had abetted the crimes. Several of the thirty-eight were political workers or involved in politics. Later, many claimed the accusation was a conspiracy to frame them.

2000-2002

On September 2, 2000, the Special Court in Kottayam found 35 of the thirty-nine accused persons guilty, while four were acquitted. Three of the convicts were women. One of the defendants died during the trial, and two others remained at large. The verdict was 356 pages long. The court criticised the police for handling the case in the early stages and their attempt to shield the accused. Various charges, including sections 120(B) (criminal conspiracy), 376(2)(B) (gang rape), 365 (kidnapping with intent to confine), and 366(A) (kidnapping with intent to rape) of the Indian Penal Code, were proven against various individuals. The sentencing took place on September 6th.

Adv. Dharmarajan was apprehended in Karnataka on September 16, 2000. He had been missing for four years. The trial of the main accused, Adv. Dharmarajan, began in 2002. On July 10, 2002, a court presided over by J. P. Chandrasekhara Pillai found him guilty of several charges, including gang rape and abduction. The court stated that as a lawyer, he was aware of the consequences of his actions, and Judge V. Chandrasekharan Nair sentenced him to life in prison on July 12, 2002. Sections 120 (B) (criminal conspiracy), 363 (kidnapping), 366 (A) (kidnapping with intent to rape), 368 (illegal confinement), 332 (hurting a public servant), 373 (buying a minor for sex), 376 (rape), 376(2)(B) (gang rape), and 392 (robbery) of the Indian Penal Code were found against him.

Adv. Dharmarajan filed an appeal with the Kerala High Court, which was denied on June 13, 2002. He only served a portion of his sentence after receiving it. On July 13, 2002, he was transferred to the Poojappura Central Prison, and on October 25, 2002, he was released on bail. After that, he vanished. Because the police could not locate him, the warrant was dropped in 2010. He had served 2 years and 92 days in prison, including pre-trial detention.

KERALA HIGH COURT VIEW

The court ruled that there was no kidnapping of a girl who had been taken by accused #1, #2, and Adv. Dharmarajan. The girl had given away her hostel fees and pawned her jewellery, but the court found no evidence of non-consent. She had been expelled from Mount Carmel School, Kottayam, and was home-tutored for a year before joining Little Flower Girls High School, Nallathanni. The court also noted that the girl's father kept a close look on her movements and frequently called the nuns of the convent school.

The girl was kept at lodges, hotels, and hospitals during her ordeal but did not attempt to escape. On 17 January, she was taken to the Kottayam bus stand, where she was taken to Ernakulam. An accused left her alone in a room for half a day without making an attempt to escape. From 22 January to 25 January, she was at the house of an accused in Vanimmel, Kozhikode. A neighbour saw her on verandas and courtyards, but she did not try to escape.

On 21 February, she was taken to Periyar Hospital in Kumily for pain in her private parts and pus coming out of her vagina. However, the doctor at the hospital said she looked normal and had a normal gait. She did not tell the doctor about her plight or her real name. On 25 February, she was staying overnight with an accused and complained of stomach pain. She was taken to Appu Hospital in Elappara, where she was diagnosed with constipation and undressed by a nurse for an enema. The robbery charge against Adv. Dharmarajan was dropped as the police could not find the ornaments.

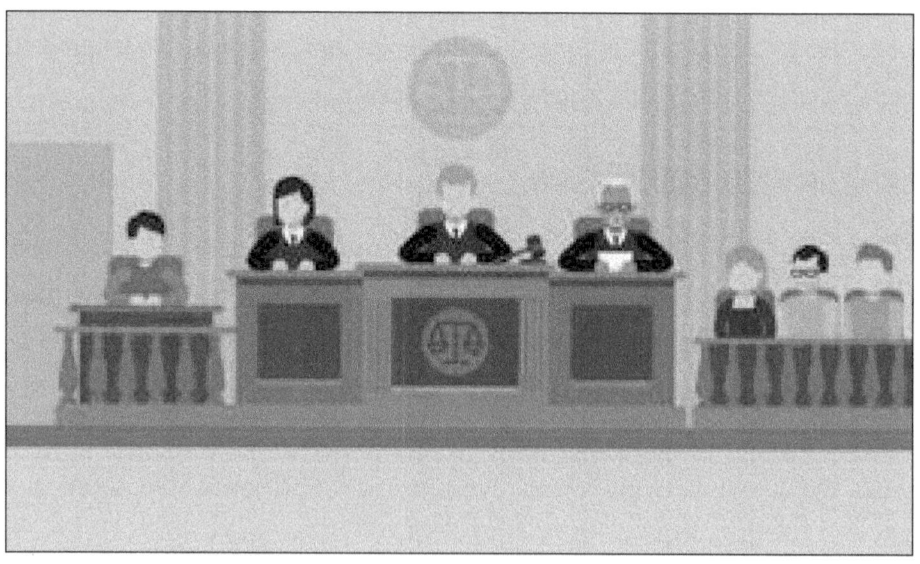

CONCLUSION

The Supreme Court of India ruled that the family could have known that Prof. P. J. Kurien was not named as an accused from media sources, leading to no cause for the delay in filing the complaint. The court also questioned why Mr. Poulose, Mr. Rajappan, and Mr. Kunjukutty were not given to the police as witnesses by the family for one year. The court found that the prior acquaintance of Mr. Poulose with the father was suspicious and that the lower court had erred by letting the case go so far.

In November 2007, a Supreme Court bench rejected an appeal from the state government seeking a retrial against Prof. P. J. Kurien but stated that it was a private complaint and no new evidence had been found. He was represented by advocate Mr. Arun Jaitley, which later became controversial. Following the 2012 Delhi rape case, a women's rights group, Janadhipatya Mahila Association, petitioned the Supreme Court of India, pointing out that the appeal against the Kerala High Court's acquittal had been pending for eight years. In January 2013, a bench set aside the Kerala High Court's order, and a fresh hearing was ordered. On April 4, 2014, a Kerala High Court bench upheld the lower court's sentence for the prime accused Adv. Dharmarajan, of life imprisonment, acquitted seven of the accused and sentenced the remaining accused to 13 years imprisonment with a fine. In case of default, it was 3 months of rigorous imprisonment. Five of the thirty-five accused died.

FUTURE PERSPECTIVES

This case would have benefited from the cops' correct work from the start. The victim's attempt to conceal or falsify certain aspects resulted in a reaction directed only at herself. The political effect on the case was significant, which caused it to lag considerably.

SOURCES & REFERENCES

- https://en.m.wikipedia.org/wiki/Suryanelli_rape_case.

Chapter 13

RAPE CRIMES AND SEXUAL VIOLENCE: CASTE AND RELIGION

Pravin N. K, Roshin F. V, and Sridhar M

ABSTRACT

This study looks at how caste and religion are connected to sexual violence cases. We explore society's rules, unfair treatment, and victims' sufferings. We also look at the problems that police and the legal system face when they deal with these cases. Understanding how caste and religion play a part in rape cases is important for coming up with good ways to stop sexual violence and make sure all the victims get justice.

KEYWORDS

Mrs. Bilkis Bano - religion-based discrimination - Gujarat - Hathras - gang rape - Uttar Pradesh - caste-based discrimination - victim's rights - marginalised communities

INTRODUCTION

Rape crimes are deeply concerning and miserable issues that impact individuals regardless of their caste, religion, or social background. These crimes are not only a violation of an individual's physical integrity but also an assault on their dignity, autonomy, and human rights. In this discussion, we will delve into the disturbing reality of sexual violence with a specific focus on how it intersects with issues of caste and religion. By exploring the interconnection of sexual violence and social factors like caste and religion, we can better understand the broader context in which these crimes occur and work toward a more inclusive society that actively condemns and prevents sexual violence in all its forms.

CASE STUDIES

CASE #1 - THE HATHRAS GANG RAPE CASE

On 14 September 2020, at around 9:30 am, the victim and her mother went to work in the fields of Boolgarhi village, Hathras district. They were working in the fields of Thakur villagers. The mother heard her screaming and rushed to find her. When she found her, she saw her lying on the ground, covered in blood, with her tongue cut off. They then took the victim to the nearest police station.

An hour later, the victim, her mother, and her brother reached the police station. The family alleged that the police deliberately delayed registering an FIR and had also told them to take the victim away. The victim's brother stated that Mr. Sandeep, one of the accused, attempted to kill her. An FIR was filed against accused, Mr. Sandeep under Section 354 of the Indian Penal Code.

SECTION 354 IPC - "Assault or criminal force to woman with intent to outrage her modesty"

The 19-year-old girl was taken to a district hospital, where the doctor referred her to the AMU JNMC Hospital due to a lack of infrastructure. She was then admitted to JNMC Hospital in Aligarh, where she stayed for 14 days, and her health continued to worsen.

The Dalit girl's statement was recorded where she alleged that she was raped by four men - Mr. Sandeep, Mr. Ramu, Mr. Lavkush, and Mr. Ravi. In her three recorded statements, she mentioned that "she was raped" and was strangled when she attempted to resist. On 29 September, the victim died of fractures and mutilations. The victim was cremated during the night at about 2:30 am by Uttar Pradesh Police without the consent or knowledge of the victim's family. The brother of the victim alleged that it was done without the family's consent and that they were locked up in their house.

When the news broke out initially through social media, Agra Police, Hathras District Magistrate, and UP's Information & Public Relations called it "fake news". Later, a senior UP Police officer claimed that **no sperm was found in samples as per the forensic report** and that some people had manipulated the incident to stir "caste-based tension." The officer also said that the forensic report revealed that the victim was not raped.

EVIDENCE TAMPERING - INVESTIGATION

The CBI began its investigation on 10 October, amid nationwide outrage, after notification from the central government. After the CBI filed a chargesheet accusing the four upper caste men of rape and murder, Hathras police arrested the four accused - Mr. Sandeep, Mr. Ramu, Mr. Lavkush, and Mr. Ravi on charges of attempt to murder, gang rape, and **violations of the Scheduled Caste and Scheduled Tribe (Prevention of Atrocities) Act, 1989.** Three of the four men accused in the 2020 Hathras case were set free by an Uttar Pradesh court Thursday. The fourth suspect, Mr. Sandeep Sisodia, was found **guilty of culpable homicide not amounting to murder** and under sections of the SC/ST Act but not of rape, reports indicated SECTION 299: - Culpable homicide.

Culpable Homicide Not Amounting to Murder

1. Provocation

2. Right of Private Defence

3. Public servant surpassing his power

4. Sudden fight

5. Consent

THE TRIAL

The trial court noted that there was **no medical evidence** of the victim's gang rape and apart from that, she had not disclosed the commission of the offence in her initial statement to the police. Moreover, the court underscored that the victim was alive until 7-8 days after the incident and was capable of talking; therefore, it could not be said that the intention of the accused was to murder her. Accordingly, the court held Sisodia guilty under Section 304 of the IPC instead of Section 302 of the IPC.

SECTION 302 OF IPC - Punishment for Murder. SECTION 304 OF IPC - Punishment for Culpable homicide.

The court said that it was the statement of the victim's mother that the victim had told the names of all the four accused and had described the incident of gang rape after two to three days of the incident.

However, this evidence was not credible as five days after the incident, the victim in her statement to the police accused only one person without any mention of rape.

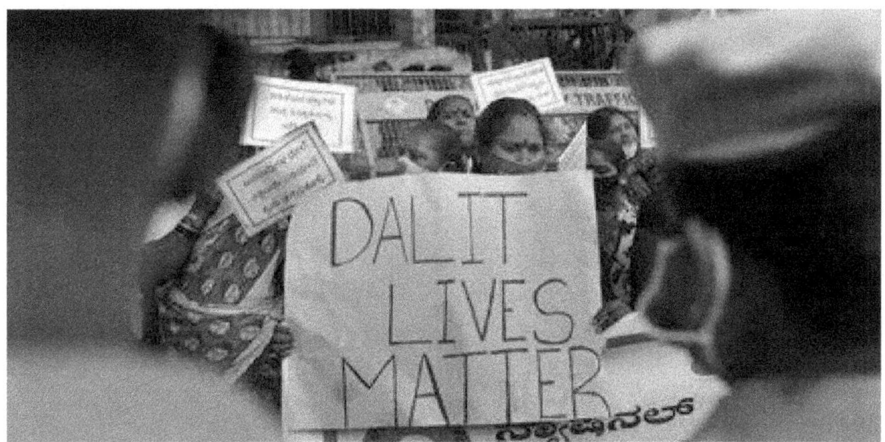

CASE #2 - THE Mrs.BILKIS BANO GANG RAPE CASE

Five months pregnant, Mrs. Bilkis Bano was 21 years old when she was brutally gang raped. This was during her attempt to flee along with her relatives in the violence that broke out during the post-Godhra communal riots in Gujarat. The mob that attacked the group killed her three-year-old daughter, Saleha, and fourteen other members of her family.

In the book **'Between Memory and Forgetting: Massacre and the Modi Years in Gujarat'**, author Mr. Harsh Mander narrates the horror. The family was moving in a truck to a village, but before they could reach their destination, a mob of 20-30 people attacked them. The men snatched the three-year-old from Mrs. Bilkis and smashed her head to the ground. With her daughter dead, three men, all belonging to her village and people she knew, took turns to rape Mrs. Bilkis. "In the mayhem around her, the fourteen members of her family were raped, molested, and hacked to death by the mob," the author notes. Taking her for dead, the assailants left her naked and unconscious. However, Mrs. Bilkis Bano lived to narrate the brutality of the heinous crime.

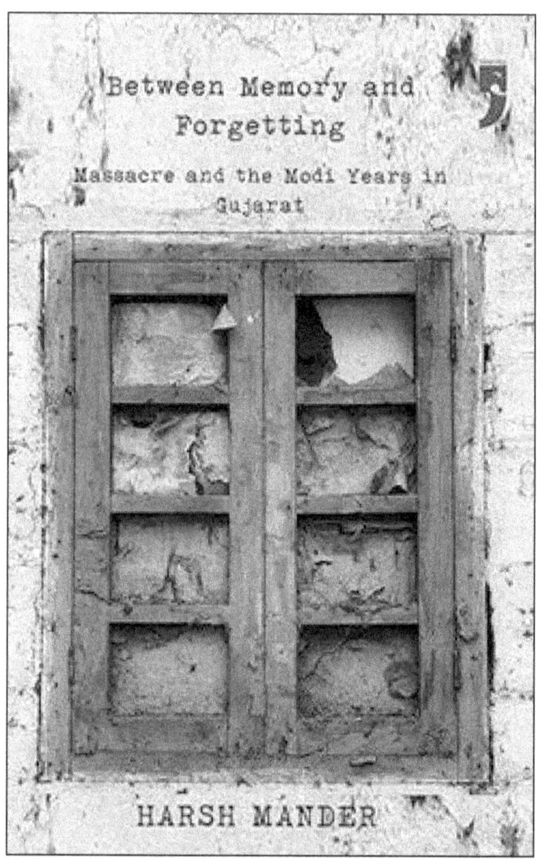

Between Memory and Forgetting:
Massacre and the Modi Years in Gujarat
—Mr.Harsh Mander

THE TRIAL AND THE JUDGEMENT

Mrs. Bilkis regained consciousness hours later, and that was the beginning of a long struggle for justice and dignity. The state machinery reportedly worked against her as she tried to get the local police to file her complaint. Even after an FIR was filed, it allegedly omitted crucial details. Mrs. Bilkis Bano approached the National Human Rights Commission (NHRC) and moved to the Supreme Court. In December 2003, the SC ordered a CBI probe into the case. A month later, all the accused were arrested, and the trial began. In August 2004, the trial was moved to Mumbai after Mrs. Bilkis Bano told the court that her family was living in the shadow of danger and uncertainty.

Four years later, the trial court found 13 of the twenty accused guilty. Of them,

1.   11 were awarded life sentences for their heinous crimes.

2.   Seven others were acquitted for lack of evidence.

3.   A three-year sentence of imprisonment was awarded to the cop who had initially refused to file Mrs. Bilkis Bano's complaint.

In May 2017, the Bombay High Court upheld the conviction and life imprisonment of all eleven and quashed the acquittal of seven others. **"I want justice, not revenge. I want my daughters to grow up in a safe India,"** Mrs. Bilkis Bano had then said. The Supreme Court later ordered the Gujarat government to pay Mrs. Bilkis Bano a compensation of Rs fifty lakh along with a job and accommodation.

THE DAWN OF INJUSTICE

As India celebrated the 75th anniversary of Independence on Monday, 11 men sentenced to life imprisonment for the gang rape of Mrs. Bilkis Yakub Rasool and the murder of seven of her family members during the 2002 Gujarat riots were released from jail in Godhra. As the eleven convicts, who walked out of the prison after 15 years, were welcomed with sweets and garlands, the Gujarat government said it relied on its old remission policy of 1992 to approve their applications for remission of the sentence and not the current policy of 2014.

'We rape to enjoy the sense of feeling dominant, not for sexual satisfaction.' This statement was given by a rapist.

CONCLUSION

Rape cases involving caste or religion are deeply concerning because they connect gender-based violence with social bias. These incidents emphasise the urgent need for legal and societal changes to fight discrimination and safeguard victims' rights. In the end, these cases remind us of the importance of building a society so that everyone can live without any fear or discrimination, and the people who commit such crimes are held accountable. It is our shared responsibility to strive for a fair and inclusive society where gender-based violence and prejudice are not tolerated.

FUTURE PERSPECTIVE

- To tackle this issue effectively, it is vital to make sure that the justice system is fair, unbiased, and responsive to survivors.
- Providing basic awareness about Article 15 among society.
- Spreading awareness about the rights and dignity of all people, no matter their caste or religion, is crucial in preventing such terrible crimes.

SOURCES & REFERENCES

- https://en.wikipedia.org/wiki/2020_Hathras_gang_rape_and_murder
- https://www.thehindu.com/news/national/other-states/dalit-girl-gangraped-by-upper-caste-men-in-   uttar-pradeshs-hathras-dies-in-delhi-hospital/article32721406.ece

- https://timesofindia.indiatimes.com/india/rape-survivor-moved-to-delhi-spine-damage- permanent/articleshow/78375589.cms
- https://www.thehindu.com/news/national/hathras-gang-rape-opposition-parties-demand-resignation-   of-up-chief-minister-yogi-adityanath/article32734523.ece
- https://www.livemint.com/news/india/Mrs.Bilkis-bano-case-supreme-court-raps-gujarat-govt-over-   selective-remission-to-accused-11692358925982.html
- https://www.civilsdaily.com/news/what-is-Mrs.Bilkis-bano-case/

Chapter 14

MS. CHRISTINE RAPE CASE-UNSOLVED

Bala Sankar. T and Devyouga Kumar. S

ABSTRACT

Ms. Christine, a 16-year-old girl from Lapu-Lapu City, Cebu, Philippines, was found murdered on March 11, 2019. Her face had been destroyed with acid, and her body had been stabbed multiple times. The police initially suspected Mr. Jonas, a man who had killed a 62-year-old man in the same way 11 months earlier. However, Mr. Jonas had an alibi for the time of Ms. Christine's murder. The police then turned their attention to Ms. Christine's 17-year-old ex-boyfriend, John. They arrested John based on CCTV footage that showed him walking with Ms. Christine on the day she disappeared. However, John's mother claimed that he was with his friends at the time of the murder. A second autopsy revealed that Ms. Christine had been killed by three other people. The police realised that John could not have been the sole killer. They also discovered that John did not have a drug habit, which contradicted the doctors' findings. John admitted destroying

Ms. Christine's face because he was inspired by the Momo challenge trend. The police are still investigating Ms. Christine's murder.

KEYWORDS

Ms. Christine Lee, Mr. Jonas, John, Blackmagic Community.

INTRODUCTION

Lapu-Lapu City is one of the largest cities in Cebu, Philippines. In that city, a 16-year-old girl named Ms. Christine was living with her mother. Ms. Christine was studying 9th grade and very calm in character both in school and at home. Ms. Christine loves to go to church often. She was attributed for her helping nature as Ms. Christine used to arrange seats for church functions. On March 10, 2019, since it was Sunday, she went to church with the permission of her mother with a condition of returning home earlier. Around 4:00 pm in the evening, Ms. Christine left for the church. Usually when she leaves for church, she will return within an hour, but that day she did not return even after 6:00 as her mother started to panic. Ms. Christine did not return home even after 7:00. So immediately her mother went to the church searching for Ms. Christine. There she asked everyone around, but they said that she had left the church early. Subsequently, she filed a missing complaint to the police.

INVESTIGATION

Police also started searching everywhere, including the places where the girl usually visits. Even after searching in most of the places, they were not able to find Ms. Christine on that particular day. On March 11, 2019, the next day after Ms. Christine went missing, early in the morning a group of people gathered in a ground. The police immediately reached the body of a teenage girl on the ground. Since Ms. Christine was missing, the police personnel insisted Ms. Christine's parents identify the body. The already grieving parents grew more concerned as it was their daughter, Ms. Christine, who was lifeless. To worsen the situation, the condition of their daughter was disheartening as her face and voice box were devastated. The body was identified by her birthmarks as her appearance was mercilessly destroyed by a homicide. Her ears, lungs, and tongue had disappeared. The body was taken for the autopsy after the confirmation.

KILLER'S ARROGANCE

At first, he had poured acid on her face so that he could peel her skin with a sharp object. The hairs on the front were plucked off, and the skin was peeled. Since the skin was peeled, all the face bones were visible outside. The appearance of the face looked horrible, like a skeleton in the Momo challenge image. Beyond all this, another brutal thing was, Ms. Christine was alive when the killer poured acid on and peeled the skin, according to the autopsy reports. The cause of death (COD) was due to strangulation of the neck, stomach, hands, and legs. She was stabbed more than thirty times with a sharp object. She had been undressed below her waist and was raped before being killed. The reason for the brutal killing of a 16-year-old girl was unknown. To get a clearer picture, the body underwent another autopsy.

PURSUIT OF PREDATOR

On the other side, police started the investigation. Surprisingly, in the same city exactly 11 months ago, a 62-year-old person was killed in the same way. Hence, the previous record of crimes was checked to find a similar kind of execution. The police confirmed that the killing style is the same and the killer might be the same too. People were furious since the 16-year-old girl did not deserve this; they started raising a voice of justice for Ms. Christine. Everyone doubted that it might be the people of the black magic community. The next day, that is on March 12, police found the killer who killed the 62-year-old person. His name was Mr. Jonas, and as people thought, he was a member of the black magic community. So, police started investigating him, thinking that he must have killed Ms. Christine, but he started giving an unexpected answer. He said to the police, "I killed the 62-year-old person, but I have nothing to do with Ms. Christine's murder." He also told that he was at a different place at the time when the murder happened. The police were perplexed to hear this and did not trust him, but during the inquiry on the day of the murder, he had really worked in other places. He had a strong alibi for his statements. The owner, under whom he had worked, confirmed that Mr. Jonas was at his place working with him on that particular day. Nevertheless, Mr. Jonas was sent to jail for killing that 62-year-old person.

THE PLOT THICKENS

The police took Ms. Christine's mobile phone into custody and started checking whether they could get any lead in that. Interestingly, an unexpected lead was found on the day when Ms. Christine disappeared, someone sent her a message on Facebook, and that message was deleted after a while. When the police investigated that person, they came to know that it was Ms. Christine's 17-year-old ex-boyfriend Mr. John. So, the police found his house and knocked on the door. John opened the door and was frightened to see the police. Immediately police arrested him and started interrogating. He said that he had nothing to do with this and he had no grudge against Ms. Christine. He firmly stated that he did not kill Ms. Christine.

On the day of the incident, Ms. Christine went to church, and it was recorded that she was walking around 6:12 in the evening. Ms. Christine did not go alone; it was recorded that a teenage boy was walking beside her. When they compared the height and shape of the body in the picture with Mr. John, it perfectly matched. According to John's mother, he went to play with his friends and was nowhere around Ms. Christine. However, he did not have any solid proof as his alibi. Since his statements were not normal, the police decided that Mr. John was the killer. So, without investigating this case further, on March 19, they closed the case. After that, a big turn and twist came in this case. The report of the second autopsy came out, and in that report, an unexpected result was waiting for the police. When Ms. Christine was murdered, by looking at the wounds from when she fought, there was no chance for the killer to be a single person. Doctors strongly said that three people were involved in this.

CONCLUSION

At the same time, people who saw Ms. Christine said that she was with three people. The investigation started again when the police were in an agitated state. Earlier, police thought that they had found one and still two more need to be found. After this result, the police even doubted whether John is the killer or not. Doctors said that at the time of the murder, the killer was high on drugs, but when they conducted a drug test on John, the result was negative. That means it was clear that John had no habit of taking drugs. Next, when the police asked why he horribly destroyed Ms. Christine's face, he answered, "In 2018, a lot of things were trending on the internet, and particularly the Momo challenge trend was being shared on the internet as a hoax. Inspired by this trend, he said that he destroyed her face." At the same time, when Ms. Christine's mom was searching for her, she might not even dream that her daughter was being fed by human creatures. Strangers are always dangerous. Ms. Christine thought that she was cheating on her mom, but she was the one who got cheated.

SOURCES & REFERENCE

- https://en.wikipedia.org/wiki/Murder_of_Christine_Silawan

Chapter 15

SIBLINGS' MURDER CASE

Priyanka E. S., Valantena M., and Anu Vasundra M.

ABSTRACT

The shocking murder of two school children, 10-year-old girl Ms. Muskan Jain and her brother, 7-year-old Master Hritik Jain, by their car taxi driver Mr. Mohan Raj and his friend in Coimbatore on October 29, 2010. These two siblings were abducted by the car taxi driver and his friend with the intention of money, but later, due to the fear of being caught, these innocent children were dumped in the PAP canal, Angalakurichi, Pollachi near Coimbatore district. Ten-year-old Ms. Muskan Jain was brutally raped before her body was dumped along with that of her brother, Master Hrithik Jain. After nine days of the murder, the accused Mr. Mohan Raj was shot dead by the allied police in an encounter, whereas Mr. Manoharan faced trial in the Mahila Court in Coimbatore in November 2012. He was given a double death sentence, three life terms after the court found him guilty of the offences alleged against him.

INTRODUCTION

This case caught attention all over Tamil Nadu, in every tea shop and home. In fact, after this incident, the black film sheets on car windows were prohibited by the government because of visibility issues.

On October 29, 2010, a horrible incident happened in Coimbatore which not only horrified the people of Coimbatore but also the people in the whole state and nation. In Coimbatore, Rangai Gounder Street, Mr. Ranjith Kumar lived with his wife Ms. Sangeetha. He was running a business, a textile shop, and the couple had a 10-year-old daughter Ms. Muskin Jain and 7-year-old son Mr. Hrithik Jain. Both were studying in a private school at Gandhipuram when their life was going normally and happily like every other child. On October 29, 2010, as the day was busy as usual in Coimbatore, Mr. Ranjith Kumar went out of town for business purposes, and both his children were getting ready for school as part of their everyday routine. They never thought that they were going to face human creatures that day. They thought it was a usual day and would return home safe, but the children were not alive when they came back home. Only their corpses were back home.

THE CASE

On 29th of October 2010, the time was exactly 7.50 a.m. in the morning. Ms. Muskin and her brother Mr. Hrithik took their lunch bag to get ready for their school. Mr. Ranjith Kumar and Mrs. Sangeetha had privately arranged for a cab from a company named "Surya" to pick the children up from the main road of their area. Usually, both the mother and grandmother accompany the kids to their cab. However, on the day of the tragic incident, an Omni van had come to pick the children up instead of the privately arranged cab. The parents were not doubting Mr. Mohan Raj (the prime convict) as he had been dropping the kids at the school regularly. Minutes after their departure, the usual cab arrived as the kids were not present; the driver questioned Mr. Ranjith about the kids' whereabouts.

Mr. Ranjith Kumar was bewildered as he informed the driver that the kids had already boarded the cab. After analysing the happenings, the parents were sure that their kids were kidnapped. On the other side, the cab was moving towards Coimbatore to Pollachi Road. Ms. Muskin had suspected something and questioned the driver about the change in the usual route, but the kidnapper had convinced her stating that it had been declared as a holiday for them, so he was taking them for a tour nearby. The unusual route had frightened the poor children as they had started to cry out of fear, but the driver had ignored the little kids' sufferings. In the next 45 minutes, the van reached Pollachi and moved toward Valparai. At the same time, Mr. Ranjith Kumar had informed the Police about this incident.

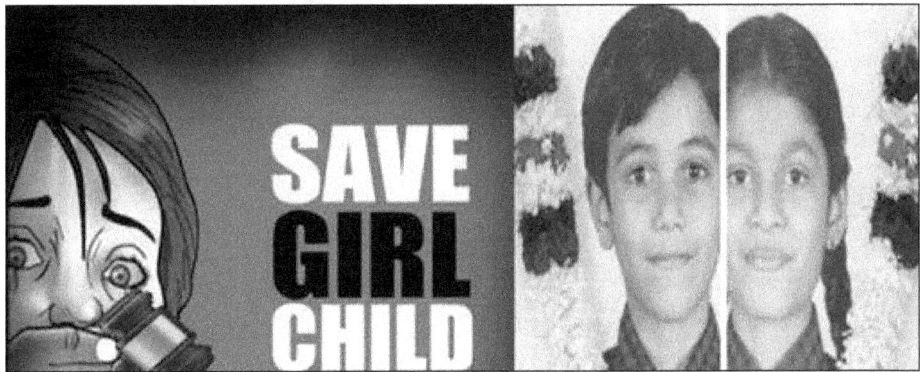

The case reached Mr. Shailendra Babu, the Commissioner of Police in 2010. Through the city police co-intelligence team, he had ordered them to check every vehicle passing through the check post. It was of no use because they had been searching for the kidnapping van, but it had already crossed Angalakurichi in Pollachi-Valparai Road. The driver of the Omni van had stopped in front of a house which belonged to an old lady. He had asked whether Mr. Manoharan was present. The old lady had replied that he was not at home.

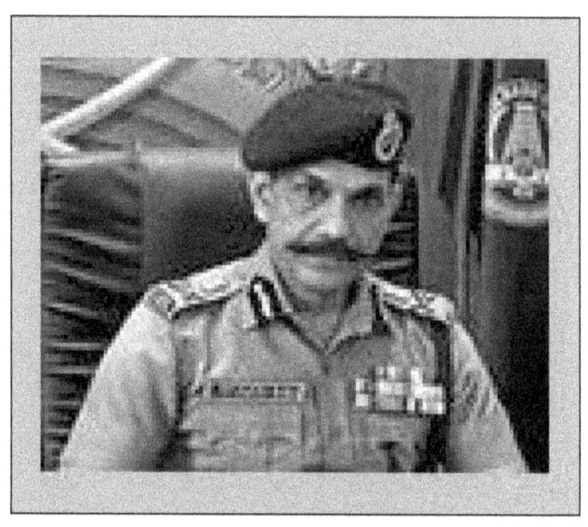

Mr. Shailendra Babu

The kidnapper had contacted Mr. Manoharan to meet him. Mr. Manoharan and Mr. Mohan Raj had taken the kids away from the city and had planned to threaten Mr. Ranjith Kumar with his kids for their own financial gain. Mr. Mohan Raj had been bankrupt as he had received a loan from the bank to own a cab. He had planned to kidnap the children and get money from their parents by threatening them for his finances. The police finally concluded that it had been a perfectly pre-planned kidnap for the purpose of their financial gain. The kidnapper had set up a caller ID on the kids' home landline so they could communicate. However, they did not receive any calls as expected. So, Mr. Mohan Raj had abruptly changed his plan of obtaining money; instead, he decided to rape and kill the school-aged child to save himself.

They had decided to rape the 10-year-old girl without any mercy. First, they had tied the hands of Mr. Hrithik and Ms. Maskin with a rope, and they had pushed Mr. Hrithik to the back side of the van. They had kicked Mr. Hrithik without any ounce of guilt. There had been a black colour sun film covering the window of the van. The happenings inside the van were not visible outside. If there was no black film in the van, someone might have saved them, and they might be alive today. The screaming and the sufferings of the children had not been heard by anyone.

The kids had already been on the verge of passing out. To escape, Mr. Mohan Raj had planned to kill both the kids. They had covered the kids' heads with a polythene cover which had made the kids suffocate.

On the way towards Anaimalai-Pazhani Road, the kidnappers tried to kill the kids, but they were unsuccessful. They had a fear that the police might locate them as they were not masters in murder. They came up with another plan to kill the kids by pushing them from the top of a mountain. By God's grace, since there was a huge crowd, the plan of killing the kids by pushing them from the mountain also went in vain. In Udumalapet, they had almost reached Deepalpatti where they had forced the kids to drink the poisoned drink. Surprisingly, the kids were smart enough to escape from the near death.

The time was exactly 10 am and the fear of the police locating them grew. In Deepalpatti, there was a big canal named PAP canal, where they stopped their car. After untying the knot of both kids, they had blackmailed the kids to eat so that they would let them free. The children refused initially, but they were forced to eat one or two chapatis after which they were beaten and kicked the 10-year-old girl, Ms. Muskin, to satisfy their desires. They threatened them to wash their hands in the canal; the kids, not knowing the consequences, washed their hands in the running water only to be pushed into the canal by the two criminals. The canal was huge; even a lot of adults had died there while bathing. Seeing the children struggling, they confirmed that they were dead. While leaving, they threw the school bag into the surroundings without knowing that it was also evidence of their brutal crime.

No sooner had the local people seen the school bag in a suspicious setting than they decided to inform the police regarding this tragic incident. The police received the information around 11.30 am; immediately, the police insisted on a search inside the canal. Disappointment was evident on everyone's face as the body of 10-year-old Ms. Muskin was found inside the canal, but Mr. Hrithik's body was nowhere to be found.

Everyone believed Mr. Hrithik to be alive. At 5:00 p.m., the police had tracked Mr. Mohanraj's phone signal, which had been near Udumalpet. Things had picked up as they arrested Mr. Mohanraj along with Mr. Manoharan. Mr. Hrithik's body had also been found on the same day. After being caught, the kidnappers confessed to their murders. There were no words to explain the pain of the parents who lost both their children. After the standard procedures, Mr. Shailendra Babu mentioned that any sort of missing cases must be reported immediately to the police so that they can proceed with the case at the earliest. In this case, the commissioner had mentioned that he was notified only at 10:45 a.m., but the kids were missing since 7:45 a.m. and had stated that if they had been informed earlier, they might have alerted the checkpoint, and things might have been better. The commissioner was also sorry for their parents as he believed that the police department was also responsible.

Then a lot of people started rising voice against Mr. Manoharan and Mr. Mohanraj after getting to know the siblings' murder case. The government got pressure from every side, including the politicians, actors, and the common people. After adjourning Mr. Mohanraj and Mr. Manoharan to the court, the Police had started the investigation separately for both of them. Unexpectedly, on the way to the court where both of them were taken separately, Mr. Mohanraj had taken the Police gun suddenly and had started threatening the driver to move towards Kerala. After a series of blasting bullets, as a result of self-defence, the police had encountered Mr. Mohanraj. After the release of the news, the public started celebrating by bursting crackers, and a lot of appreciation was given to the commissioner.

Mr. Manoharan did not know about the encounter of his partner. Realisation hit him after knowing the encounter of his partner. He got terribly scared that he might also lose his life. The police completed the investigation in 45 days as they filed a 400-page crime report in the Women's High Court. 126 witnesses were investigated along with eighty-five documents. The judgement was given in 2012, as it was proved that Mr. Mohanraj and Mr. Manohar were found guilty. As a punishment for Mr. Manoharan's gruesome rape, he was given three life sentences and two death sentences. The common people celebrated the judgement given by the court.

Now to save himself, Mr. Manoharan's lawyer had appealed for an amendment in the final verdict given by the court, but the High Court turned down the appeal. Three days before the final penalty, the Supreme Court ordered to stop the penalty for Mr. Manoharan. The court had also favoured Mr. Manoharan by insisting the court revise the petition given to him. After several disagreements and disapprovals, in 2019, Mr. Manoharan was given the death penalty for committing the unforgivable crime. The date for the death penalty was not fixed, and Mr. Manoharan was alive in jail as of 2019.

CONCLUSION

The incident had evoked a public outrage where people threw eggs on Mr. Mohanraj when he was brought to the court. Soon after their arrest, the students and teachers of Coimbatore had elucidated wearing black badges and holding prayers on the day of cremation of the victims. After this incident, the black film sheet in car windows had been prohibited in Tamil Nadu. Such an incident created a great impact on society. An awareness programme regarding laws related to children's safety should be conducted, and children must also be aware of these (Child helpline number in India: 1098).

It is disheartening to even think about the agony the children had undergone. The judgement given by the court can never bring those innocent souls back, but it would be apprehensive for the perpetrators living in this society.

SOURCES & REFERENCES

- https://www.thehindu.com/news/cities/Coimbatore/coimbatore-siblings-murder-case-supreme-court-confirms-death-penalty/article28787313.ece
- https://timesofindia.indiatimes.com/city/chennai/coimbatore-twin-murder-girl-was-raped-by-driver/articleshow/6849541.cms
- https://www.ndtv.com/india-news/execution-of-man-who-murdered-2-tamil-nadu-siblings-stopped-by-top-court-2102366

Chapter 16

THE ASSASSINATION OF MR. RAJIV GANDHI

Rohith Sugu S, Bitto K, and Beula M

ABSTRACT

At least one national government, the Inder Kumar Gujral administration, was overthrown by conspiracy claims that were investigated by two commissions of inquiry. The former Indian Prime Minister Mr. Rajiv Gandhi was killed on May 21, 1991, in Sriperumbudur, Tamil Nadu, India, by a suicide bombing. There were at least fourteen other people who died in addition to Mr. Rajiv Gandhi. The 24-year-old Kalaivani Rajaratnam, a member of the Tamil separatist organisation Liberation Tigers of Tamil Eelam (LTTE), which is outlawed in Sri Lanka, carried it out. In addition, she goes by the aliases Dhanu and Thenmozhi Rajaratnam. During that period, India had just used the Indian Peace Keeping Force to withdraw from the Sri Lankan Civil War.

KEYWORDS

Mr. Rajiv Gandhi, Dhanu, LTTE, Tamil Eelam, assassination, transvaluation.

PICTORIAL REPRESENTATION

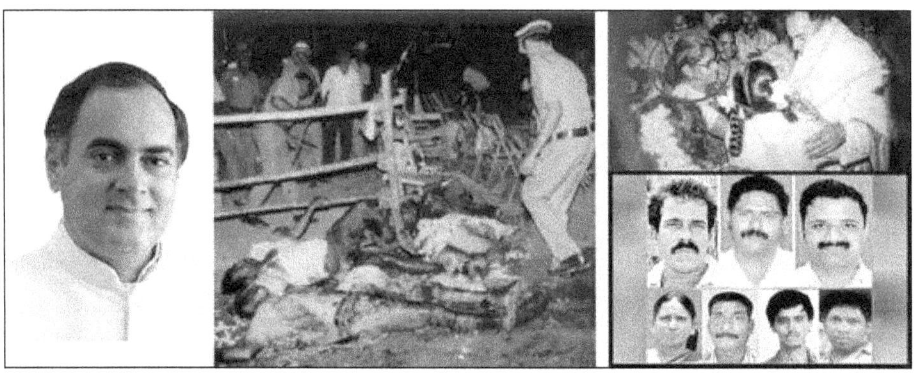

ASSASSINATION

Mr. G.K. Moopanar and Mr. Rajiv Gandhi were hard at work managing election campaigns in the southern Indian states. On May 21, after concluding his campaign trail at Visakhapatnam, Andhra Pradesh, he moved on to Sriperumbudur, Tamil Nadu. After landing in Madras (now Chennai), Mr. Gandhi was driven to Sriperumbudur by a motorcade in a white Ambassador automobile, stopping along the way at a few other places where election campaigns were being held. The trip took around two hours. Mr. Rajiv drove up to a campaign event in Sriperumbudur, got out of the car, and walked over to the dais where he was supposed to speak. Along the journey he was showered with flowers by many well-wishers, including school children and members of the Indian National Congress. The assassin, Ms. Kalaivani Rajaratnam, approached and welcomed him. Then, at exactly 10:10 p.m., she bent to touch his feet and detonated a belt that was concealed beneath her clothing and contained RDX explosives. Following the explosion, forty-three people were seriously injured and Mr. Gandhi, his assassin, and fourteen other individuals died. Mr. Hari Babu, a local photographer who also died in the explosion, caught the assassination on camera. His film and camera were found unharmed at the scene.

VICTIMS

Apart from the suicide bomber Ms. Kalaivani Rajaratnam, twelve persons lost their lives in the explosion that occurred on May 21, 1991: the following people were present: Mr. Rajiv Gandhi, the former prime minister; Dharman, a police constable; Santhani Begum, the leader of the Mahila Congress.

- Mr. Rajguru, a police inspector
- Mr. Chandra, a police constable
- Mr. Edward Joseph, a police inspector
- Mr. K.S. Mohammed Iqbal, the superintendent of police
- Ms. Latha Kannan, a Mahila Congress worker, who was accompanied by her daughter Kokilavani
- Ms. Kokilavani, the ten-year-old daughter of Latha Kannan, who sang a poem to Gandhi just before the blast
- Mr. Darryl Jude Peters, an attendee and observer
- Mr. Munuswamy, a former member of the Tamil Nadu Legislative Council
- Ms. Saroja Devi, a seventeen-year-old college student
- Mr. Pradeep K Gupta, Rajiv Gandhi's personal security officer
- Mr. Rafaelhandran, the Black Cat commando
- Mr. Murugan, a police constable

The explosion also injured about forty-three onlookers, including the police sub-inspector Ms. Anushiya Daisy.

INVESTIGATION

Shortly after the assassination, on May 22, 1991, the Chandrasekhar government handed over management of the investigation to the CBI. The agency formed a special investigation team under the direction of Mr. D. R. Karthikeyan to identify the assassin. The confirmation of the LTTE's involvement in the murder by the SIT probe was endorsed by the Supreme Court of India. According to the commission report from 1989, "the perpetuation of the general political trend of indulging the Tamil militants on Indian soil and tolerance of their wide-ranging criminal and anti-national activities." The inquiry also asserted that LTTE leaders in Jaffna were privy to confidential, coded communications that were exchanged between the union and state administrations. Evidence points to the interchange of some of the most significant wireless signals.

PERPETRATOR

Ms. Kalaivani Rajaratnam, also known as Dhanu, was the assassin. On July 26, 1968, she was born in Kaithady, Nunavil, on the Jaffna Peninsula. She became known by the assumed name Thenmozhi after joining the LTTE. Her family was from the little Jaffna village of Kupukullai. She attended Batticaloa and Vavuniya schools. Additionally, she briefly resided in Urumpirai. At an early age, she was inspired by the Tamil militant group Liberation Tigers of Tamil Eelam, also known as the Tamil Tigers, and following an ankle injury, she joined the Black Tigers, a group of suicide bombers. She carried the flag for female LTTE marches and was referred to as "captain Akino." Mr. A. Rajaratnam, a Tamil man from Sri Lanka, and his second wife were Kalaivani's parents. Mr. A. Rajaratnam's first wife died in 1962 while he was touring tea estates. Rajaratnam, who was Velupillai Prabhakaran's mentor, was reported to have had a profound impact on the leader of the LTTE's thinking between 1972 and 1975, when the movement was still in its early stages. Kalaivani was only 7 years old in 1975 when A. Rajaratnam passed away. After his body was removed from Chennai, his funeral was held in Jaffna. At the time of her death, Kalaivani's marital status was unknown to the public. Kalaivani was survived by his mother, brother Mr. Sivavarman, and two sisters, Anuja and Vasugi, the latter of whom was killed in combat with the Indian army. Two of the plot's co-conspirators, Mr. Sivarasan and Ms. Subha, have ties to Kalaivani. While Sivarasan's mother, Sivapackiyam, was Kalaivani's father's sister, Subha's parents are related to Sivarasan's father. Since many of them had drastically different front and side profiles, it was also believed that the Rajaratnam-Pillai dynasty's genetics may have played a role in their selection for the Rajiv Gandhi assassination. The seven individuals who helped arrange Rajiv Gandhi's assassination were found guilty and given life sentences.

Six convicts in the 1991 Rajiv Gandhi assassination case were ordered to be released by the Supreme Court of India on November 11, 2022, in response to the government of Tamil Nadu's controversial recommendation for their remission in March 2016. The prisoners are:

- Mr. Murugan, also known as Sriharan, is a Sri Lankan LTTE agent.

- Ms. Nalini, Murugan's wife. Nalini is an Indian national.

- Mr. Santhan, also known as T. Suthenthiraraja, is a citizen of Sri Lanka.

- Mr. Robert Pious is a citizen of Sri Lanka.

- Mr. Jayakumar: Robert Pious's brother-in-law.

SUPREME COURT JUDGEMENT

Judge Mr. K. T. Thomas of the Supreme Court of India ruled that Rajiv Gandhi's decision to send the Indian Peace Keeping Force (IPKF) to Sri Lanka and the IPKF's purported atrocities against Sri Lankan Tamils were personal grievances held by Prabhakaran, the leader of the Liberation Tigers of Tamil Nadu (LTTE). The killing resulted from this animosity. In addition, the Rajiv Gandhi administration incited PLOTE and other Tamil militant organisations to topple the military coup in the Maldives in 1988. The death of Mr. Thileepan during a hunger strike and the suicide of 12 LTTE cadres aboard a vessel in October 1987 were also included in the verdict.

Even though several other Indians were slain, the verdict found no proof that any of the conspirators ever wanted the killing of any other Indian, even though four of the accused were found guilty and given death sentences. Judge Wadhwa went on to say that there was no evidence in the file indicating that the goal of killing Mr. Rajiv Gandhi was to subdue the government. As a result, it was decided that the Terrorist and Disruptive Activities Act (TADA) did not classify it as a terrorist act. Judge Thomas went on to say that the plan was hatched over several years, starting in 1987. When the decision to kill Rajiv Gandhi was made could not be determined by the special investigation team of the Central Bureau of Investigation, the top special investigation agency in India.

TRIAL

The legal foundation for the Mr. Rajiv Gandhi assassination trial was established by the Terrorist and Disruptive Activities Act (TADA).

The problem started in 1998 when all twenty-six suspects were given death sentences by the TADA court in Chennai. Legal professionals and human rights organisations criticised the trial for not meeting the standards for a fair trial. The accused later claimed that their confessions to the Superintendent of Police were obtained under duress, which formed the basis of their conviction.

CONCLUSION

Following an appeal to the Supreme Court, only four of the defendants received the death penalty; the other accused received different prison sentences. Nalini Sriharan, one of the accused, was the only survivor of the assassination group. Rajiv Gandhi's widow Sonia Gandhi intervened in 2000 and managed to have her death sentence lowered to life in prison. In 2011, the death row inmates Murugan, Santhan, and Perarivalan requested clemency, but their request was turned down by the Indian President. In response to their pleas, the Madras High Court postponed the execution, which was scheduled for September 2011, for a duration of eight weeks. Nalini also asked for parole after serving for more than 20 years, but the state government rejected her request. The three convicted men insisted that they were political prisoners rather than common criminals.

SOURCES & REFERENCES

- https://www.britannica.com/biography/Rajiv-Gandhi
- https://www.inc.in/our-inspiration/shri-rajiv-gandhi
- https://images.app.goo.gl/NVbEegCQs1zB8Srn7

Chapter 17

THE BLACK WIDOW OF KERALA – CYANIDE JOLLY

**Swetha A, Sri Janani G, Abishek W. J.,
Beritto Jackson, and Joel K. John**

ABSTRACT

Ms. Jolly Joseph, also known as the "Black Widow of Kerala," is responsible for the six murders that happened in 14 years at Koodathayi, a small village in Kozhikode district, Kerala. This case is also known as the Koodathayi cyanide murders. The cause of death of the five victims - Ms. Annamma Thomas, Mr. Tom Thomas, Mr. Roy Thomas, Mr. Mathew Manjayadil, and Mr. Sily Shaju - was cyanide poisoning, and the 6th victim, Mr. Alpine Joseph, was killed by choking on food.

KEY WORDS

Cyanide Jolly – Cyanide Poison – Koodathayi Murders – Black Widow of Kerala – Koodathayi Cyanide Poison

INTRODUCTION

Ms. Jolly Joseph (Jollyamma) was from Kuttappana, Idukki district in Kerala. In 1997, she was married to Mr. Roy Thomas and had two sons. Ms. Jollyamma was believed to be an M.Com graduate and had a job at the National Institute of Technology. The family of Mr. Roy Thomas (Thomas Family) was very rich, and all the authority of the house was in the hands of her mother-in-law, Annamma Thomas. When Ms. Jolly found that Ms. Annamma Thomas was bossy over her, she decided to kill her. In 2002, Ms. Annamma Thomas was poisoned to death. After Ms. Annamma's death, the authority of the house was now in the hands of Mr. Tom Thomas (Jolly's father-in-law). So, she decided to kill him. In 2008, Mr. Tom Thomas was also poisoned and passed away. Then she decided to kill her husband, Mr. Roy Thomas, and in 2011, she poisoned him by mixing it with the food, and his body was found inside the bathroom, which was locked from inside, and thus the police stated this as a murder. Mr. Mathew Manjayadil (brother of Annamma Thomas) grew suspicious about the three deaths in the family, and he requested the police for a post-mortem report of Mr. Tom's body. Mr. Jolly became alert as she would be accused if the results of the post-mortem report were released. To safeguard herself, she decided to kill Mr. Mathew Manjayadil.

In 2014, Mr. Mathew Manjayadil was killed. Ms. Jollyamama had an affair with Mr. Shaju Zacharia (cousin of Roy Thomas), and he also had a family. Since it was disturbing her own life with Mr. Shaju, she killed Ms. Alphine Shaju (daughter of Shaju) in 2014, and in 2016 she killed Ms. Sily Shaju, the wife of Mr. Shaju Zacharia. Ms. Jollyamma then married Mr. Shaju Zacharia in 2016. In 2018, Mr. Rojo Thomas (son of Annamma) read the autopsy report of his brother Mr. Roy Thomas. He found that the statement by Ms. Jolly and the autopsy report were not the same. He suspected Ms. Jollyamma may be the killer. In 2019, Ms. Jollyamma was arrested with two others, Mr. M S Mathew (jewellery shop owner) and Mr. Praji Kumar (Goldsmith), who were also involved by providing her with the poison (potassium cyanide).

THE CASE

Early Life

Ms. Jollyamma, also known as The Black Widow of Kerala, was from Kuttapana, Idukki, Kerala. She belonged to a very good family; she was very good at her academics, and she owned a charity and was into social work with church members. According to her neighbours, she was pretty and was a professor at the National Institute of Technology, Calicut. Ms. Jollyamma got married to Mr. Roy Thomas in 1997 and had two sons (Mr. Romo Thomas and Mr. Roland Thomas). After marriage, Ms. Jollyamma lived together with her father-in-law and mother-in-law in Koodathayi, Kozhikode, Kerala. Thomas's family was very rich as most of the family members were teachers and government staff; they had a big house and owned multiple pieces of land in their area. Their family had ten members, and they lived together as a joint family. Mr. Tom Thomas and Ms. Annamma Thomas were the elders in the family; they had two sons (Mr. Roy Thomas and Mr. Rojo Thomas) and one daughter (Ms. Renji Thomas). Mr. Tom Thomas had a brother (Mr. Zacharia Thomas); he had a son, Mr. Shaju Zacharia. Mr. Shaju was the cousin brother of Mr. Roy Thomas. Ms. Annamma Thomas had a brother, Mr. Mathew Manjayadil. Roy Thomas was living with his parents, and Mr. Rojo Thomas was in the US for his studies and job. He also owned a house in the US and visits India once a year.

THE FIRST VICTIM IN THE THOMAS FAMILY

At first, Ms. Jollyamma was happy with her new family, but later when Ms. Jollyamma found that Ms. Annamma was suspicious of her studies and her fake job, she also had an eye on the property because her husband's family was very rich. The pride and the authority of the property were with Ms. Annamma Thomas, mother-in-law of Ms. Jollyamma. After a year of her son's birth, with the permission of her family, she joined her work and later joined NIT as a commerce staff, but soon her mother-in-law became very strict and restricted her freedom. She found that Ms. Annamma would be a problem for her to attain the property and have control over her freedom. So, she decided to kill her. On 22-08-2002, when Ms. Annamma came back to the house after a walk, she gave her a bowl of mutton soup which was mixed with potassium cyanide. After drinking this, Ms. Annamma felt dizzy and stumbled. She fell in front of the house while walking. Later she was taken to the hospital, and on the way to the hospital, Ms. Annamma died. Doctors stated that it was a heart attack, and the whole family also believed it because she was getting older. Later her body was buried in a cemetery in Lourdes Matha Church, located near Koodathayi.

TWO MURDERS, FOUR YEARS

She had the next hindrance in her path, Mr. Tom Thomas (Father-in-law), was then the head of the house and she also decided to kill him. Mr. Tom Thomas was sixty-five when he died; he was a strong man physically and did physical exercises every day, but on that day, Mr. Tom had not done any exercises and he was feeling very weak because he ate boiled tapioca, which was mixed with poison. This happened when Ms. Jollyamma and Mr. Tom were alone in the house. Later, he collapsed in the room and was taken to the hospital, where he also died on the way. Although the deaths of Ms. Annamma and Mr. Tom Thomas were exactly the same, the family members thought he also died because of a heart attack on 26-08-2008. The doctors also did not reexamine the cause of Mr. Tom's death as he was already ageing. He was buried next to Ms. Annamma Thomas.

Her next target was her husband, Mr. Roy Thomas, who was working as a distributor in a private company. Since he had a loss in his business, he started working as an oil and petroleum distributor. Ms. Jollyamma already had an affair with Mr. Shaju Zacharia (cousin brother of Mr. Roy Thomas), and she also wanted to marry him. On September 9, 2011, she gave him rice and curry which was mixed with potassium cyanide. Mr. Roy ate the food by 8:30 pm (says the autopsy report) but Ms. Jollyamma told everyone that he had never eaten the food after 3 pm. Soon after eating, he felt dizziness and on the way to the hospital, he died. Thus, the third death in the house has occurred, but the weirdest part is that every death happened in the same way. The police stated that it was a suicide because he was found dead inside the bathroom, and they said that he might have committed suicide by consuming poison because of financial problems. Ms. Jollyamma requested everyone not to talk about his suicide to escape from her own pre-planned murders.

TWO MURDERS IN ONE YEAR

Mr. Mathew Manjayadil, the uncle of Mr. Roy Thomas and brother of Ms. Annamma Thomas, had doubts about the three deaths that happened in the family one after the other in the same manner. He started arguing about this, and the whole family started convincing him, but he was not convinced and asked for Mr. Tom's autopsy report.

According to him, old people might die because of natural causes, but how could the same thing happen to Mr. Roy when he was not old too? So, he requested a detailed autopsy report. Later, fear started arising for Ms. Jollyamma because if he gets the autopsy report, he will uncover her dark secrets. To avoid this, she kills Mr. Mathew Manjayadil by giving him poisoned coffee. This incident occurred on February 24, 2014.

Later, after the death of Mr. Roy, Ms. Jollyamma had more interactions with Mr. Shaju Zacharia. She visited him frequently after Mr. Roy's death, but there was a problem in marrying Mr. Shaju as he had a family and a child of his own. Ms. Alphine Shaju was the daughter of Mr. Shaju Zacharia and Mr. Sily Shiju who passed away at the age of two. The cause of her death was due to choking on food which was given by Ms. Jollyamma. She killed Ms. Alphine because if Ms. Alphine was there, then Mr. Shaju would have sympathy towards his daughter and eventually he would not accept to marry Ms. Jollyamma. This made her kill the 2-year-old baby. Ms. Alphine was the only one in the family who did not die of a heart attack. One fine day, Ms. Jollyamma was invited to attend the First Holy Communion at Mr. Shaju's house. She went earlier to his house and started involving herself in cooking for the guests. She fed Ms. Alphine Shaju bread, which choked her, leading to her death on 3rd May 2014. The post-mortem of the body was not taken as she already had an asthma problem and had been receiving treatment since her birth.

THE LAST VICTIM

Ms. Sily Shaju, the wife of Mr. Shaju Zacharia, was the last victim of Ms. Jollyamma. She killed Ms. Sily because she needed to marry Mr. Shaju Zacharia. On January 11, 2016, when Ms. Sily was in the dental clinic, Ms. Jolly gave water to Ms. Sily, and she died on the spot with excessive froth in her mouth. In the same year, after some weeks of Ms. Sily's death, Mr. Shaju Zacharia and Ms. Jollyamma got married. This marriage was approved by her family as she told her family that she needed another marriage, and the family members also accepted her wish as Ms. Jollyamma was in her thirties only during her second marriage.

THE COMEBACK OF ROJO

Mr. Rojo, the brother of Mr. Roy and the son of Mr. Tom Thomas and Ms. Annamma Thomas, who was in the US, came back to his native country when he heard about the six mysterious deaths in his family. He was suspicious about Ms. Jollyamma because, after the third day of Mr. Roy's death, she had gone on a tour with her colleagues. Then Rojo asked for the autopsy report of his brother Mr. Roy Thomas. On seeing the report, he found out that his brother had died of poison and the last food he ate was rice and curry at 8:30 pm, but Ms. Jollyamma said that Mr. Roy had not taken any food after 3:00 pm. This increased his doubts about her. Then Mr. Rojo Thomas filed an RTI (Right to Information) application with state authorities. At the same time, Mr. Rojo tried to find out about Ms. Jollyamma's job details and found that everything was a lie, that Ms. Jollyamma did not have a job at NIT. She had visited the beauty parlour shops and spent her time gathering in the canteen at NIT. On investigating her to the college authorities, they said that they had not seen her, and she was not a member of staff working in the college. Mr. Rojo had a strong doubt on her because soon after Mr. Tom Thomas and Ms. Annamma Thomas's death, she sent a will to him (Rojo), and before the death of his father (three months prior) the entire property of the house and the lands were changed to Ms. Jolly's name. These reasons also made him feel that Ms. Jollyamma was the suspect, and the investigation started again.

THE INVESTIGATION AND ARREST

The investigation of the Koodathayi Cyanide murder Case was held by rural SP Mr. Simon in October 2019. This led to the arrest of Ms. Jollyamma and two others who helped her in this series of murders. Then the reports were sent to different Forensic Science labs, and it was found that traces of potassium cyanide were present on the bodies of the victims. On further investigations, it was found that Ms. Jolly had poisoned her husband Mr. Roy Thomas to death. It was also found that the will which was changed to Jolly's name was forged by Ms. Jollyamma. Then on October 05, 2019, she was arrested for murdering her first husband (Roy Thomas). She also confessed that she had committed all six murders for the sake of property. The two others who were arrested along with Ms. Jollyamma were Mr. Prajikumar (the goldsmith) and Mr. M S Mathew (the jewellery shop owner). Mr. M S Mathew was a jewellery shop owner who lived near the house of Ms. Jollyamma and helped her by providing the necessary poison. He had obtained poison from Mr. Prajikumar by offering him two bottles of alcohol and 5000 rupees as a bribe. Mr. Prajikumar used potassium cyanide for cleaning jewellery items. Ms. Jollyamma asked for poison in the name of killing the rats in her house. Based on the above reasons and evidence, the three people were arrested.

OTHER PLAYERS IN THE CRIME

I.   RETIRED SUB-INSPECTOR

Mr. Ramanunni was in charge of Kodenchery police station. He classified the death of Mr. Roy Thomas as an alleged suicide, even though the report had revealed traces of potassium cyanide in his body.

II.   REVENUE OFFICIAL

A lady tahsildar, Ms. Jayashree, helped Ms. Jollyamma to prepare a fake will.

III. IUML LOCAL LEADER

A Muslim League leader who was in frequent contact with Ms. Jollyamma helped her to transfer her father-in-law's property to her name.

IV. CPI(M) MEMBER

Mr. Manoj, a CPI(M) leader, signed as a witness for the fake will after receiving one lakh rupees from Ms. Jollyamma.

V.   A CRIMINAL LAWYER

He was a frequent visitor to Ms. Jolly's house after the death of her husband, Mr. Roy Thomas.

VI. A BSNL EMPLOYEE

He was found to be in regular touch with Ms. Jollyamma, usually at night.

PICTORIAL REPRESENTATION

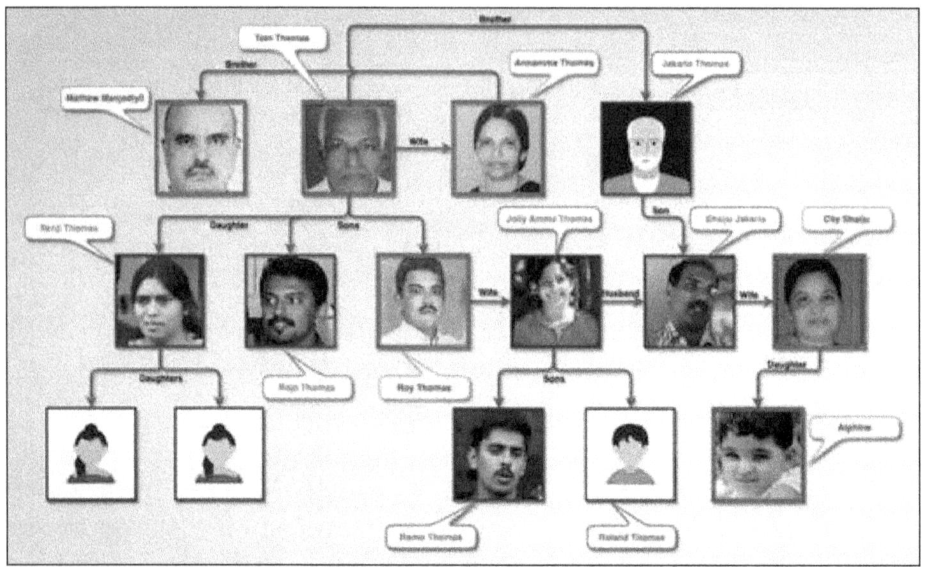

The Family tree

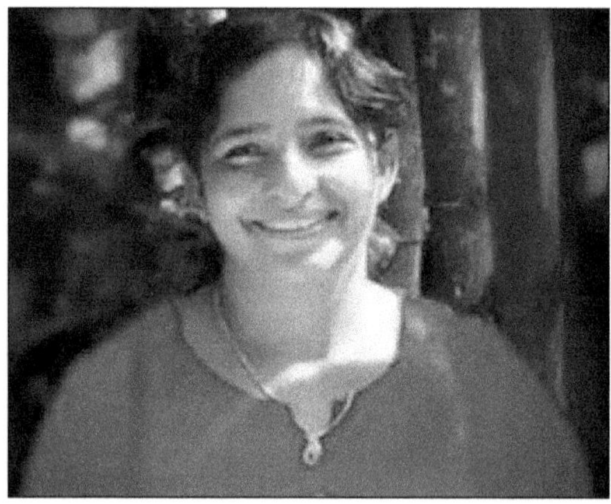

Jollyamma

TABLE

SNO	NAME OF VICTIM	CAUSE OF DEATH AND YEAR	RELATIONSHIP
01	Ms. Annamma Thomas	Died on 22-08-2002 after consuming poison-mixed mutton soup given by Jollyamma.	Mother-in-law of Jollyamma.
02	Mr. Tom Thomas	Died on 26-08-2008, after eating poison-mixed boiled Tapioca which was given by Jollyamma	Father-in-law of Jollyamma.
03	Mr. Roy Thomas	Died on 09-09-2011 after eating poisoned rice and curry cooked by Jollyamma.	First husband of Jollyamma.
04	Mr. Mathew Manjayadil	Died on 24-02-2014 after drinking poisoned coffee given by Jollyamma.	Brother of Annamma
05	Ms. Alphine Shaju	Died on 03-05-2014, from choking on food that was fed by Jollyamma.	Daughter of Shaju (Jolly's second husband).
06	Ms. Sily Shaju	Died on 11th January 2016, after drinking water that was given by Jollyamma.	Shaju's First Wife

CONCLUSION

In this case, the greed of Ms. Jolly over the property of the Thomas family led to the death of the six members. One of her victims was just two years old. For fourteen years, death appeared to have been stalking the members of a family, and the main reason for death was cyanide poisoning according to the forensic report taken during the second post-mortem under the FIR of Mr. Rojo Thomas, the brother of late Mr. Roy Thomas. The cases became serious because of the suspicious death of the two-year-old Ms. Alphine as it was not possible for a baby to have a heart attack at the age of two years. All those deaths had one detail in common, and that is, Ms. Jollyamma was present at every incident as a fake wife and had a fake job during her 17 years of life. She faked herself to attain all the properties and to live with the love of her life, Mr. Shaju Zacharia, the cousin of Mr. Roy Thomas.

FUTURE PERSPECTIVE

Ahead, we are aware of such a case of Ms. Jollyamma, the highly reactive chemical which is harmful to human beings should not be distributed without any legal authentication in the chemical utility store. More action should be taken as a precaution. Promoting more towards mutual understanding marriages, so that there should not be any contempt for each other, unlike in Ms. Jollyamma's case. Each deceased person, whether old or young, should be sent for a post-mortem. People working in chemical industries must have a regular weekly or monthly check-up since there might be a slight presence of chemicals which can cause slow poisoning later.

SOURCES & REFERENCES

- http://surl.li/mfzbt
- http://surl.li/mfzcb
- http://surl.li/mfzch
- http://surl.li/mfzcq
- http://surl.li/mfzcw

Chapter 18

UNMASKING THE GOLDEN STATE KILLER: SOLVING A DECADE-OLD MYSTERY

Raju Nandhakumar

ABSTRACT

The Golden State Killer, also known as the East Area Rapist and the Original Night Stalker, was a prolific serial killer and rapist who operated in California from 1974 until 1986. He committed at least thirteen murders, nearly fifty rapes, and numerous burglaries. The assailant primarily targeted suburban neighbourhoods, breaking into homes at night. For decades, the case remained unresolved, perplexing the investigators despite DNA evidence. In 2018, a former police officer named Mr. Joseph James DeAngelo was arrested when investigators utilised genetic genealogy to connect his DNA to the crime scenes. Mr. DeAngelo eventually pleaded guilty to the crimes in 2020, averting the death penalty by accepting a life sentence without parole. His arrest and conviction were a breakthrough in cold case investigations, highlighting the potential of emerging forensic tools like genetic genealogy in solving decade-old crimes.

KEYWORDS

Genetic genealogy, Burglaries, Law enforcement, Cold cases

CASE BACKGROUND

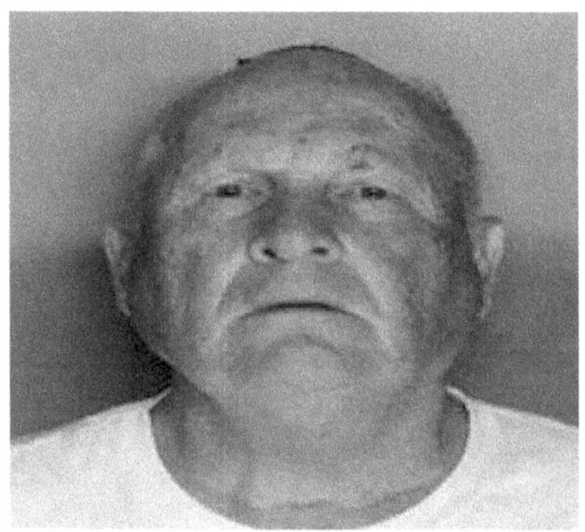

Mr. DeAngelo - The Golden State Killer

THE GOLDEN STATE KILLER'S MODUS OPERANDI (MO)

The Golden State Killer meticulously planned and stalked victims, conducting detailed surveillance of their homes. He made harassing phone calls and returned to some victims' homes. Initially targeting women alone or with children, he later targeted couples, demonstrating growing violence and audacity. He targeted people in their homes during the early morning hours. Mr. DeAngelo was known for breaking into homes by prying open windows or cutting through screens, using weapons like knives or guns, and using physical restraints like ties and items found in the victims' homes such as towels or belts, to bind or restrain them. He blindfolded and gagged his victims to prevent them from seeing or screaming for help. The Golden State Killer was known for psychological manipulation, separating couples by tying up the male victim, placing dishes on his back, and threatening to kill both victims if the dishes made noise while he assaulted the female. He also committed sexual assaults, often over several hours, leading to more brutal attacks and eventually murder. His level of violence escalated over time.

FIRST MURDER IN 1979

The Golden State Killer was a notorious serial killer who systematically robbed victims' homes, often stealing sentimental items. He also exhibited bizarre behaviours, such as eating food from their refrigerators or taking breaks during the assaults. Initially, his attacks did not lead to murders, but his violence escalated over time, leading to his murders. Mr. Brian and Ms. Katie Maggiore were killed in Rancho Cordova in 1979, which was his first known homicide. His lack of physical evidence at murder scenes helped him evade detection for years.

ESCAPE AND TAUNTING LAW ENFORCEMENT

The Golden State Killer was a meticulous and calculated criminal who often evaded detection by walking through neighbourhoods, parks, or drainage ditches. He would spend extended periods in victims' homes, ensuring they were too terrified to move or call for help. His ability to evade capture for decades demonstrates his knowledge of law enforcement techniques, possibly influenced by his experience as a former police officer. His careful planning, control over his victims, and evolving violence made him one of the most feared criminals in California. His ability to shift his motive over time made it difficult for law enforcement to connect the various crime sprees, until DNA evidence finally connected them.

MAJOR BREAKTHROUGH

In 2018, advancements in DNA technology and genetic genealogy led to a breakthrough in the Golden State Killer case. During the 1970s and 1980s, DNA technology was not advanced enough to identify the killer, but biological samples from crime scenes were preserved. As DNA testing improved, law enforcement began connecting crimes committed by the East Area Rapist and the Original Night Stalker, revealing they were dealing with the same person. Traditional DNA databases, like Combined DNA Index System (CODIS), did not match the killer's DNA profile, causing the investigation to stall. In 2018, investigators turned to genetic genealogy, uploading the killer's DNA profile to publicly available genealogy websites like GEDmatch. These sites allowed people to upload their own DNA to trace family heritage or find relatives. Investigators used these databases to find distant relatives of the Golden State Killer, narrowing down possible suspects through genealogical research.

Investigators identified Mr. Joseph James DeAngelo, a former police officer, as the suspect in the Golden State Killer case. They used genealogical research to identify family members who shared enough DNA with the killer, leading to the identification of Mr. DeAngelo. Other circumstantial evidence, such as Mr. DeAngelo's age, location, and history, also matched the timeline and geography of the crimes. In order to verify the match, they watched Mr. DeAngelo and took a discarded sample of DNA. When the DNA was compared to the crime scenes, a precise match was discovered. Mr. DeAngelo, at the age of 72, was taken into custody at his Citrus Heights, California, home on April 24, 2018, after it was discovered that his DNA matched that of crime locations. Earlier, his experience in law enforcement during the crimes likely helped him avoid capture.

GENEALOGY AND DNA TECHNOLOGY

1. DNA Profiling

DNA collection: The Golden State Killer case involved DNA samples collected from crime scenes in the 1970s and 1980s, preserved by law enforcement despite the lack of technology for full analysis at the time.

DNA Matching: In the late 1990s and early 2000s, law enforcement utilised DNA profiling techniques to link multiple crimes, such as identifying the East Area Rapist and the Original Night Stalker through matching profiles.

CODIS (Combined DNA Index System): Traditional law enforcement databases like CODIS contain DNA profiles of arrested or convicted individuals, but the Golden State Killer's DNA did not match anyone in these databases due to his lack of a serious crime history.

2. Genetic Genealogy

As consumer DNA testing services like Ancestry.com and 23andMe gained popularity, people began uploading their DNA to private companies to trace their ancestry or find relatives. These companies provide users with their genetic profiles and allow them to connect with biological relatives through shared DNA segments. GEDmatch, a public platform, was used in the Golden State Killer case to compare and build family trees, unlike private companies, which were accessible to law enforcement for investigations.

3. Confirming the Match

In 2018, law enforcement uploaded the DNA profile from the Golden State Killer crime scenes to GED match, aiming to locate distant relatives whose DNA partially matched the crime scene DNA. Genealogists worked with law enforcement to build family trees using historical records, obituaries, and other genealogical data to trace these relatives back to a common ancestor and modern-day descendants. This process narrowed the suspects to Mr. Joseph James DeAngelo, who fit the profile in terms of age, geographic location, and other characteristics. After identifying Mr. DeAngelo as a prime suspect, investigators subtly collected his DNA and compared it to the crime scene DNA, finding a perfect match. After being detained in April 2018, Mr. DeAngelo admitted to several crimes, including rapes, murders, and incidents of burglary. Subsequently, he was given a life sentence.

4. Significance of Genetic Genealogy in Law Enforcement

Numerous cold case investigations were reopened utilising genetic genealogy as a result of the Golden State Killer case, which signalled a major shift in the field. But this case brought up issues with privacy and morality around police enforcement's use of genealogy databases. DNA testing companies have since clarified their policies on accessing user data without permission. Following the case, law enforcement agencies began adopting genetic genealogy as a standard tool for cold cases, raising legal and ethical questions about privacy, consent, and the extent of genealogical data use. Advances in DNA technology and genetic genealogy have made solving decades-old crimes more feasible, and genetic genealogy has been used to solve numerous other cold cases, providing closure to families who had given up hope. Criminal investigations have changed significantly as a result of the convergence of genetic genealogy and DNA technology.

Mr. DEANGELO'S MURDERS: A TIMELINE

The East Area Rapist, a legendary serial killer, is a criminal organisation that has committed several atrocities across California.

The organisation started in 1973 with the first burglary in Visalia and went on to commit over 100 additional crimes. In 1975, the Ransacker shot and killed 16-year-old Elizabeth Hupp and her father. In 1976, the group attacked the first victim, Phyllis Henneman, and raped Kris Pedretti. In 1978, Katie and Brian Maggiore were fatally injured. In 1979, the group broke into the home of a Danville couple but managed to flee. Lyman and Charlene Smith were killed with a fireplace log in 1980, while Patrice Harrington was raped and beaten to death with a brass sprinkler head. In 1986, Janelle Lisa Cruz was raped and killed in her parents' residence. In 1997, criminalist Paul Holes unearthed old papers on the East Area Rapist and began looking into the case. When Holes compared the East Area Rapist's DNA to Mary Hong's Original Night Stalker profile in 2001, he was given the identity of "Original Night Stalker-East Area Rapist." Voters in California approved Proposition 69 in 2004, and an all-felon DNA database was created. In 2018, the FBI renewed the investigation and offered a $50,000 reward for information leading to his arrest. Joseph James DeAngelo was arrested in April 2018 and later pleaded guilty in return for a life sentence.

CAPTURE AND CONVICTION

Mr. DeAngelo was initially charged with thirteen counts of murder related to the Golden State Killer crimes, with some cases linked to rapes and other violent offences. Investigators linked the Golden State Killer to approximately fifty rapes and 120 burglaries, but the majority of these crimes were unable to be prosecuted due to statutes of limitations. Mr. DeAngelo made several court appearances, appearing frail and disoriented. On June 29, 2020, he entered a guilty plea to thirteen counts of first-degree murder and other charges, ensuring he would spend the rest of his life in prison without parole. During his guilty plea hearing, victims and their families shared powerful victim impact statements, expressing anger and relief that justice had finally been served after years.

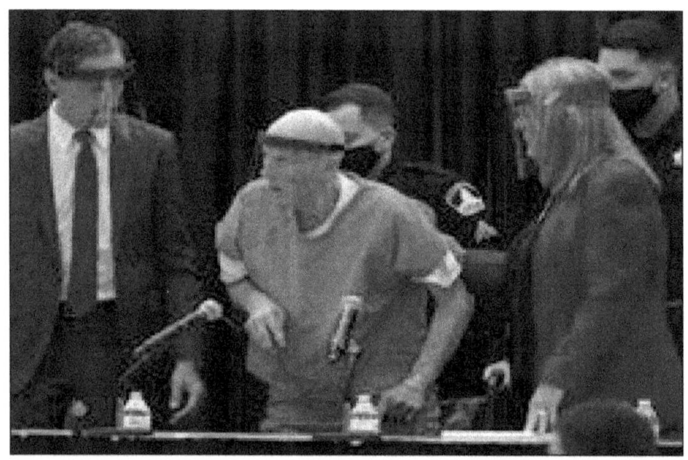

Mr. Joseph James DeAngelo pleads guilty to thirteen murders. tagged to California's Golden State Killer

SENTENCE

On August 21, 2020, Mr. Joseph James DeAngelo received a life sentence without the possibility of parole. Survivors and families of victims addressed him during a three-day hearing, describing the decades-long devastation his crimes caused. Mr. DeAngelo showed little emotion during the sentencing but apologised in a brief statement. The sentencing brought closure to many victims and their families, ending one of California's darkest chapters in criminal history.

CONCLUSION

The Golden State Killer case was one of the first high-profile cases solved using genetic genealogy, a powerful investigative technique for solving cold cases and identifying unknown suspects. This led law